Measuring Quality of Life in Health

For Seema, Suji and James

For Churchill Livingstone:

Editorial Director: Mary Law
Project Development Manager: Claire Wilson
Project Manager: Samantha Ross
Design: Judith Wright

Measuring Quality of Life in Health

Rod O'Connor BSc(Hons) CHEc PhD

Conjoint Senior Lecturer, School of Public Health and Community Medicine,
The University of New South Wales, Sydney, Australia
Executive Director, Rod O'Connor & Associates Pty Ltd

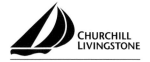

CHURCHILL
LIVINGSTONE

EDINBURGH LONDON NEW YORK OXFORD PHILADELPHIA ST LOUIS SYDNEY TORONTO 2004

First published 2004

ISBN 0443073198

British Library Cataloguing in Publication Data
A catalogue record for this book is available from the British Library

Library of Congress Cataloging in Publication Data
A catalog record for this book is available from the Library of Congress

Notice
Medical knowledge is constantly changing. Standard safety precautions must be followed, but as new research and clinical experience broaden our knowledge, changes in treatment and drug therapy may become necessary or appropriate. Readers are advised to check the most current product information provided by the manufacturer of each drug to be administered to verify the recommended dose, the method and duration of administration, and contraindications. It is the responsibility of the practitioner, relying on experience and knowledge of the patient, to determine dosages and the best treatment for each individual patient. Neither the Publisher nor the editors assumes any liability for any injury and/or damage to persons or property arising from this publication.   **The Publisher**

your source for books,
journals and multimedia
in the health sciences
www.elsevierhealth.com

The
publisher's
policy is to use
paper manufactured
from sustainable forests

Printed in China

Contents

Preface

This book is concerned with the assessment of health outcomes from the patient's perspective. Patients and their families may know the effects of ill-health and treatment better than anyone, but traditionally little formal attention has been given to outcomes as patients perceived them. Healthcare administrators and bureaucrats are concerned with process – the great machine of healthcare proceeds inexorably on. Clinicians have traditionally been concerned primarily with physiological outcomes.

Over the last few decades there has been mounting change. The need to measure people's own views regarding the experience of illness and treatment has been recognized, resulting in a host of outcome measures concerned with assessing patients' attitudes, experiences, perceptions, ability to carry out the activities of daily living, and quality of life in general.

This book is concerned with patient-centred measures. It aims to provide a perspective for understanding their range and ambitions, and to indicate the potential that measures of this type have for improving healthcare. It reveals how much is being learned about the psychological mechanisms that mediate quality of life, and the implications for future measures. More basically, the book introduces skills needed for the selection, appraisal, use and development of measures of patient-centred outcomes, and skills for measuring health as it is perceived and experienced by patients.

The book shows that we live in interesting times in health outcomes measurement. The field is expanding into exciting new areas of research. These include the way health states are perceived and experienced, new techniques for developing scientific measures, and tests that may prevent future health states and not merely describe current ones. Hopefully the book will act as a compass to negotiate these issues and assist the reader to make effective choices about measurement. Ultimately, its intention is to help healthcare workers gather information from patients so as to make better healthcare decisions.

The book discusses the background to health outcome measures and their basis in clinical medicine, health economics, and psychometrics. Questions that confront practitioners are considered such as the place of single-item global questions and when to use a generic versus a disease-specific measure. It also provides the reader with a set of criteria for assessing the adequacy of an instrument and addresses when and how to develop a new measure.

There is a need to improve the understanding of quality of life measures. This book aims to de-mystify and clarify issues, and to reveal that there is indeed 'gold in them there hills'.

Who should read this book?

This book is aimed at those involved in applying, developing, and researching measures of patient-centred health outcome, be they quality managers, administrators, or researchers. It is relevant to clinical medicine, allied health, community care, and to anyone who wishes to understand and improve health outcomes from the patients' perspective.

This book aims to give the reader the ability to:

- Explain the aim of patient-centred health outcomes measurement and how it relates to traditional healthcare measurement
- Understand the range of patient-centred measures, including health-related quality of life, functional health status, and patient satisfaction
- Recognize the key role that patients play as active agents in their own quality of life
- Specify the aim of a health measurement instrument in operational terms and know why this is important
- Explain what is meant by test validity and how to develop and assess validity
- Explain the role of test reliability and associated techniques (e.g. Cronbach's Alpha)
- Explain the relative advantages of measures based on Classical Test Theory, Rasch analysis/Item Response Theory, and single items, in measuring patient-centred outcomes

- Appreciate the distinctive origins and diverse nature of common instruments
- Critically assess an instrument
- Commence the development of a new measure for assessing patient-centred outcomes for a treatment programme or population.

Acknowledgements

The author is indebted to many people connected with the writing of this book. To mention just a few: Ken Forster for his inspiring supervision of my PhD many years ago that encouraged the idea that intellectual argument could be fun; Shane Thomas for supporting me in the idea that I might actually write this book; Trevor Bond for his comments on my interpretation of the Rasch model, and Colin Schoknecht for his good friendship and unique intelligence that has resulted in so many casual remarks becoming an occasion for whimsy, amusement, and insight. To those who I should have mentioned and haven't, please forgive me.

Abbreviations

ACSA	Anamnestic Comparative Self Assessment
ADL	activities of daily living
AMAQ	Asthma Medication Adherence Questionnaire
ANOVA	analysis of variance
AQLQ	Asthma Quality of Life Questionnaire
CAT	computer adaptive testing
CFA	confirmatory factor analysis
CHQ	Chronic Heart Failure Questionnaire
COPD	chronic obstructive pulmonary disease
CPX	symptom-problem complex
CRQ	Chronic Respiratory Disease Questionnaire
CTT	Classical Test Theory
CUA	cost-utility analysis
DIF	differential item functioning
DSP	Disability Support Pension
ES	effect size
EORTC QLQ-C30	European Organization for Research and Treatment of Cancer 'Quality of Life Questionnaire Core 30 Items'
EQ-5D	The Euroqol-5D questionnaire
FACT	Functional Assessment of Cancer Therapy
FIM FIM-SM	Functional Independence Measure
FLIC	Functional Living Index – Cancer
GP	general practitioner
HQoL	health-related quality of life
ICC	item-characteristic curve
IIRS	Illness Intrusiveness Ratings Scale
IRT	Item Response Theory
IWB	Index of Well-Being
JND	just noticeable difference

KR-20	Kuder-Richardson formula 20
MCID/MID	minimal clinical importance difference
MR	multiple regression
MSAS	Memorial Symptom Assessment Scale
MAU	multi-attribute utility
NHIS	National Health Interview Survey
NNT	number of patients needed to treat
OET	Occupational English Test
PCA	Principal Components Analysis
PCI	Prostate Cancer Index
PGI	patient generated index of quality of life
QALYs	quality adjusted life years
QoL	quality of life
QWB	Quality of Well-Being [index] [scale]
RAND-36	The RAND 36-item health survey
RCT	randomized control trial
SD	standard deviation unit
SEM	standard error of measurement
SF-6	6 item short-form survey (a subset of the SF-36)
SF-12	12 item short-form survey (a subset of the SF-36)
SF-36	Medical Outcomes Study (MOS) 36 item short-form health survey
SGRQ	St George's Respiratory Questionnaire
SIP	Sickness Impact Profile
SWB	subjective well-being
TTO	time tradeoff
VAS	visual analogue scale
WAIS	Weschler Adult Intelligence Scale
WATs	Work Ability Tables
WHOQoL	World Health Organization Quality of Life
WOMAC	Western Ontario MacMaster osteoarthritis questionnaire
1PL (2PL, 3PL)	one-parameter logistic (etc.)

Context, role and nature of patient-centred health outcome measures

---

AIMS OF CHAPTER

- To reveal the aim of patient-centred health outcome
  measurement and the factors encouraging its use
- To show that terms such as 'health-related quality of life' (HQoL)
  need to be rigorously defined when used, and that this is not
  characteristic of the literature

- To provide an overview of the range of patient-centred measures, including HQoL, functional status, patient satisfaction, and dynamic measures

OUTCOMES RESEARCH – EVALUATING THE QUALITY OF HEALTHCARE

Outcomes research – the study of the end results of health care, that take patients experiences, preferences and values into account – is intended to provide scientific evidence relating to decisions made by all who participate in health care (Clancy & Eisenberg 1998, p. 245).

Health outcomes research is fundamentally concerned with evaluating the quality of healthcare: on the one hand with assessing the effectiveness of medical programmes and healthcare services, and on the other with gathering direct evidence of whether medical treatments are beneficial for an individual patient. This direct evidence includes ability to function and quality of life (QoL). By linking the care people receive to the outcomes they experience, outcomes research is seen as the way to investigate and improve the quality of healthcare.

QoL, functional health status and patient satisfaction, are primary measures of outcome for health programmes, used increasingly when assessing the effects of disease or healthcare. These patient-centred measures aim to comprehensively assess an individual's health state or health-related experience, and characteristically investigate a broad range of aspects of perceived importance to the individual. Health outcomes research is based on such measures; as they become widespread it is increasingly important that healthcare workers can understand, assess, select and improve them.

FACTORS ENCOURAGING THE USE OF QUALITY OF LIFE MEASURES IN HEALTH

The World Health Organization (1947) defined health as 'not merely the absence of disease, but complete physical function, social function, role function, mental health and general health perceptions'. This definition signaled a change in the way that health and healthcare was evaluated, and a move to the development of patient-centred measures.

In essence, health outcome measures evolved from survival and clinical events, to patient-centred outcomes, particularly health-related quality of life or HQoL (for an overview of this history, see Wood-Dauphinee 1999).

HQoL, the most prominent patient-centred outcome measure, is now regularly included in clinical trials. In 1998, around 10% of all randomized cancer clinical trials included HQoL as the main end point (Sanders et al 1998).

Factors responsible for the development of patient-centred measures are described below.

The need to assess the relative merits of health programmes

The need to have measures of health programme effectiveness that go beyond traditional output measures (such as number of patients treated) has been a major motivation for the development of health-status assessment instruments. There has been an increasing need to allocate health service resources rationally across diverse health programmes.

Arising from this, a number of measures of the broad effects of ill-ness on a patient's life have been developed with the declared aim of assisting health policy decisions, particularly utility measures such as the Rosser index (to allow evaluation of health service funding; Gudex 1986), Torrance's health utility approach (to facilitate decisions regarding programme funding; Torrance et al 1972), and the Quality of Well-Being index (Kaplan & Anderson 1988, Kaplan et al 1989).

Even the Sickness Impact Profile (SIP), developed by Bergner and co-workers seemingly outside the context of utility theory, had this as a declared aim. Bergner stated that the SIP was developed with the specific aim of providing information on the efficacy of health programmes to assist decisions regarding the appropriate allocation of the government's resources. The aim was to provide a 'fiscally and logistically practical measure of health status' (Bergner et al 1976a, p. 393, also see Bergner et al 1976b).

The desire to comprehensively assess the impact of clinical therapies

Advances in medical research and therapy have shifted health-care resources from the diagnosis and treatment of infectious disease to the prevention and control of chronic disease: with this has come an increased emphasis on changes in functional status and QoL outcomes (Revicki 1989).

Patients now survive conditions they would once have died from, although they may be left with health states that are valued as worse than death (Heyland et al 1998). Modern treatments may also have undesirable side effects. The consequences of treatment and treatment-related side effects may affect all of a patient's life, e.g. becoming bald and nauseous, being on a restricted diet, being tied to a machine 12 hours out of 24. It is important to assess all aspects of a treatment's effects (Bergner 1989).

Medical interventions may also result in improved functional health status without evidence of physiological change, e.g. pulmonary rehabilitation programmes may improve exercise capacity without altering pulmonary function tests. Alternatively, therapy may result in physiological improvement without apparent clinical benefit, e.g. nitrate therapy may alter haemodynamics in patients with heart disease without improving exercise capacity (Deyo & Patrick 1989).

Cancer is an area particularly concerned with QoL issues. Donovan et al (1989) noted that the emotional suffering produced by cancer tends to exceed the physical suffering it causes.

The recognition that patients have a distinctive view of their health

The description and evaluation of a health state differs according to whether the patient, a doctor, or a member of the general public provides the appraisal.

The assessments of patients and doctors differ markedly

In a study examining the effects of anti-hypertensive therapy, it was found that 100% of physicians thought the patients QoL had improved following the beginning of therapy, but only 44% of the patients themselves reported feeling improvement, 44% felt no change, and 8% felt worse. At the same time assessment by relatives was that QoL had decreased for more than 90% of the patients (Jachuck et al 1982).

Substantial differences between patients' appraisals and that of their doctors was also found by Hall et al (1989). When patients were asked to give global ratings of their own health, they drew on aspects relating to emotional, functional, and physiological health. In contrast, their physicians ratings appeared to be primarily based on physiological health, with relatively little regard for emotional health. This emphasis by doctors upon physical more than psychosocial aspects was earlier reported by Martin et al (1976) when examining the SIP.

In a more recent study, the views of multiple sclerosis patients were compared to their clinicians (neurologists and neurosurgeons). Rothwell et al (1997) reported disagreement on which domains of health status were most important; patients rated vitality, general health, and mental health more highly (as defined by the SF-36) but were less concerned about physical disability.

A review of cancer studies found that clinicians often failed to stress symptoms their patients were concerned with, and suggested that patient-report questionnaires needed to become standard practice in the assessment of cancer patient HQoL (Bottomley 2002).

The separation between doctor and patient judgements may increase as the doctor becomes more senior

Estimates of patients' functional health made by first, second and third year residents and staff physicians were found to have steadily decreasing correlations with patients' total SIP scores, which was interpreted by Hall et al (1989) to reflect a steady narrowing of the physician's perspective on the patient's health. Similarly, Bergner et al (1976b) reported that the correlation between patient self-assessed SIP score and clinical rating declined with the length of time the physician had been in practice.

Patients differ from the uninformed public: the experience of the health state causes a change in its assessment

It is apparent that the experience of the health state causes a change in its assessment. A study examining the attitudes of 18 pregnant women towards anaesthesia during childbirth found that experienced mothers differed from first-time mothers in feeling more strongly about avoiding anaesthesia during as well as outside of the delivery period (Christensen-Szalanski 1984). Patients with end-stage renal disease also value life more than the public believes (Tsevat et al 1990).

Ill subjects (medical and psychiatric patients) and nurses tend to give higher magnitude valuations for severe illness states than do healthy subjects (Kind & Rosser 1988), and valuations of health states differ between healthy volunteers and patients (Sackett & Torrance 1978). Carter et al (1976) also reported that non-health workers tended to give higher ratings of dysfunction to illness behaviour statements than did health professionals and students.

Patients increasingly wish to have their views heard

The increase in attention to the views of patients and the general public may also reflect the increasing education of the population and the desire to be involved in decisions regarding their own healthcare (cf. Donaldson 2003, Kennedy 2003).

The potential benefits for clinical practice

Measures of Quality of Life are now established in clinical trials and are beginning to enter clinical practice

While introducing HQoL into oncology has been difficult, clinicians are increasingly considering the importance of HQoL in the care of cancer patients (Bottomley 2002; see also Osoba 1994, Tanaka & Gotay 1998, Bezjak et al 2001).

The impact of computer-administered QoL measurements in oncology clinics was examined by Velikova et al (2002), who found that it led clinicians to enquire more often about daily activities, emotional problems and work-related issues, with an overall increase in the number of issues discussed. Patients felt that the questionnaires were a useful tool to tell the doctors about their problems, while clinicians perceived that the QoL data helped to identify issues for discussion and to detect change over time.

QoL measures in clinical practice have the potential to ensure that treatment and evaluations focus on the patient rather than the disease, with benefits in both the clinical encounter and quality improvement (Higginson & Carr 2001), although to achieve this the appropriateness and accuracy of measures needs to be ensured and the concerns of clinicians allayed. The potential benefits include a better focused consultation, more accurate health status assessment, and more efficient use of consultation time.

Direct attention at appropriate areas – guided history taking

A potential value of QoL measures is to direct the clinician to areas of concern to the patient.

The feasibility of introducing the European Organisation for Research and Treatment of Cancer Quality of Life Questionnaire Core 30 Items (EORTC QLQ-C30), a cancer-specific QoL questionnaire, into the daily routine of an out-patient oncology clinic was investigated by Detmar & Aaronson (1998), with physician and patient receiving a copy of the summary just prior to the medical consultation. They found that the availability of the summary appeared not to lengthen the average consultation time, but that it stimulated physicians to inquire into specific aspects of the health and well-being of their patients, which both clinicians and patients saw as a benefit.

Formal QoL assessments can provide systematic, quantitative answers to the kinds of questions clinicians usually ask informally, such as 'how have you been lately?' (Till 1994). With epilepsy, Cramer (1999) suggested HQoL questionnaires can be used to assess the effects of seizures and medications on cognitive function, memory, mood, physical health, and health perceptions, and allows patients to express their concerns about a variety of diagnosis-related issues that are often not brought to the attention of the physician.

More accurate status assessment

Data from clinical trials suggest that QoL measurements may predict survival. Chang et al (1998) examined the relation between survival and QoL measurements among patients with colon, breast, ovary, or prostate cancer, using the Memorial Symptom Assessment Scale (MSAS), a patient-rated, multidimensional instrument that evaluates the intensity, frequency, and distress associated with 32 physical and psychological symptoms. They reported that MSAS physical symptom subscale score was a predictor of survival, and noted that experience in cancer pain management had demonstrated a high prevalence of inadequate assessment and that the measurement of physical symptoms and related distress via the MSAS could aid assessment the impact of cancer and its treatment. (See also Bottomley 2002, Velikova et al 2002.)

More effective consultations

There is evidence that QoL questionnaires can be used in the clinical setting without increased demand on consultation time and with more satisfied clients and clinicians (Velikova et al 2002, Detmar & Aaronson 1998). Little et al (2001) surveyed and followed-up patients attending general practitioner (GP) clinics and concluded that consultations that produce more satisfied patients result in patients with less symptom burden and less health service usage. They noted that satisfaction is important in its own right but that it also predicts compliance with treatment and medical outcomes (cf. Little et al 1997).

Greater informed choice regarding treatments

There is a need to provide evidence to patients in a way that allows them to make an informed choice. This is a potentially important area for patient-centred health outcomes research – documenting and presenting the consequences of specific illnesses and treatments in the areas that patients consider most important and in terms that are most meaningful (Haynes et al 2002, O'Connor et al 2000). This might include information on the degree to which people adapt to what might seem quite undesirable health states (Redelmeier et al 1993, and see Ch. 2).

WHAT IS HEALTH-RELATED QUALITY OF LIFE?

There is a wide range of different concepts that can be referred to when the term 'quality of life' is used in health. Bottomley (2002) reported locating the following:

- The state of well-being as a composite of both the ability to perform everyday activities that reflect physical, psychological, and social well-being, and patient satisfaction with levels of functioning and control of the disease.
- Subjective evaluation of the good and satisfactory character of life as a whole.
- The gap between the patient's expectations and achievements; the smaller the gap, the higher the QoL.
- The functional effect of an illness and its consequent therapy as perceived by the patient.

- An individual's overall satisfaction with life and general sense of personal well-being.
- Patients' perceptions of their position in life in the context of the culture and value systems in which they live and in relation to their goals, expectations, standards, and concerns. (See also Pugh-Clarke et al 2002.)

Most commonly, HQoL is taken to refer to patients' subjective experience of their overall health state, conveyed by their own reports. HQoL measures are members of a larger family of *patient-centred measures*, measures that aim to assess and/or promote health as it is experienced by patients. HQoL measures are the most numerous of this group, which includes such measures as patient satisfaction, functional status, and medication compliance.

Box 1.1   A rough guide to some terms

Health-related quality of life or HQoL. The component of QoL due to the person's health state. Most commonly refers to patients' subjective experience of their global health, but may refer to (health-related) subjective well-being, functional status, or self-perceived health. Most commonly, HQoL measures are based on patient report.

An early representative definition of HQoL is: 'a multi-dimensional concept that encompasses the physical, emotional, and social components associated with an illness or treatment' (Revicki 1989). One based on the World Health Organization definition of health states that HQoL 'includes psychological and social functioning as well as physical functioning and incorporates positive aspects of well-being as well as negative aspects of disease and infirmity' (Sloan et al 2002b).

Functional health status. Ability of the patient to carry out normal activities, or a sub-set of their normal activities. It is often observer based, but may be based on patient report.

Some describe functional health status measures as a sub-set of QoL/HQoL measures (Bowling 1997), while others see QoL/HQoL and functional measures to be clearly separable (Muldoon et al 1998).

Self-perceived health, or terms such as 'health perception'. Patients' direct report of their global health. This may be gathered using a scale with defined end points, e.g. 'rate your health on a 100 point scale, where 100 = as fit as an Olympic athlete, and 0 = perpetual coma'. It is generally based on patient report.

Patient satisfaction. The consumer's appraisal of healthcare received. It is generally based on patient report.

Quality of Life or QoL. Outward material circumstances or subjective well-being. It may refer to physical, emotional, subject-determined, or observer measures. It may or may not be based on the subject's report.

There are a large number of health-related quality of life/health status measures available

Garratt et al (2002) conducted a systematic search of electronic databases to identify work relating to patient-assessed health outcome measures: 3921 reports were located that described the development and evaluation of patient-assessed measures, with 650 new reports in 1999 (the last year surveyed). Garratt et al reported that of all articles, cancer, rheumatology and musculoskeletal medicine accounted for more than 20% and the elderly 8%, with relatively little development and evaluation of measures for burns and trauma, intensive care, and gynaecology.

They noted that it was surprising that gynaecology was so poorly developed, given that so many problems are chronic and associated with substantial psychosocial distress.

Wide variation in terminology and no common reporting method

Deyo & Patrick (1989) reported that concepts relevant to health and QoL were diverse, scattered through many disciplines, and used many different labels (e.g. health status, functional status, disability scale, quality of life). Bergner (1989) noted that the notion of QoL had been a category in *Index Medicus* since 1966, yet QoL was usually not defined in the reports of clinical trials, and 'definitions must be deduced from the dimensions assessed', and that 'each investigator that purports to address quality of life actually examines a very narrow and specific set of factors'. Generally, notions of QoL were not specified, being more inferred than explained.

Gill & Feinstein (1994) found that the situation had changed little. Of about 75 articles considered, investigators conceptually defined QoL in only 15%, identified the targeted domains in only 47%, gave reasons for selecting the chosen QoL instruments in only 36%, and aggregated their results into a composite QoL score in only 38%. No article distinguished 'overall' QoL from HQoL.

Sanders et al (1998) examined the frequency and quality of reporting on QoL in randomized controlled trials, concluding that the term 'quality of life' was often used vaguely and without clear definition, and standards for assessing and reporting QoL in clinical research trials needed to be developed. More recently, Lee & Chi (2000) located 20 cancer randomized controlled trials (RCTs) that included HQoL measures and identified major deficiencies in providing a rationale for HQoL assessment and inadequate description of methodology. See also Garratt et al (2002), Haas (1999).

Much terminology is interchangeable

In part reflecting the large number of disciplines that have an interest in the area (including clinical epidemiology, psychology, psychometrics, statistics, health economics, operations research, and artificial intelligence), there are many terms with very similar if not the same meaning.

In particular, the terms 'construct', 'dimension', 'domain', 'area', 'attribute', 'ability', 'trait', 'true score', 'factor', 'latent trait' and 'concept' can have similar meanings. All might be used to refer to the hypothetical unifying variable (or 'latent' variable) that underlies a cluster of related items. For example, the *construct* (or domain, etc.) of 'ambulation' may refer to the abstract notion of 'ability to move from one place to another unaided', represented by expressions such as 'unable to run' and 'can walk a few steps then requires to rest'.

The terms 'tests', 'instruments', 'tools', 'measures' and 'scales' form another cluster, and all may be applied to questionnaires (or possibly single items) used to measure or estimate constructs.

It needs to be pointed out that the term 'scale' can also refer to the *response options* that are provided for answering a particular item. For example, some items in a test may be answered by ticking a response on a 'Likert scale' (typically three to seven response options, e.g. 'Strongly Agree', 'Agree', 'Neither Agree nor Disagree', 'Disagree', 'Strongly Disagree'), while other items will require the respondent to place a mark on a visual analogue scale or VAS (a straight line with two labelled endpoints, e.g. 'state of perfect health' and 'coma').

Important: always define terms carefully

It is essential to determine *how terms are being used in a particular context.*

For example, when the phrase 'health-related quality of life' is used, readers need to conduct their own assessments of whether such a measure includes relevant dimensions, is based on patient report, etc.

Failing to do this could lead to falsely assumed definitions and an erroneous interpretation of results.

Within this area 'rating scale' is another term of variable meaning: it can refer to a VAS, or to a task responded to via a 0–100 rating or an ordered set of response categories *without* a pictorial representation.

THE SUBJECTIVE/OBJECTIVE CONTINUUM

Much early health status literature focused on observable behaviours, and showed little interest in patient feelings (e.g. Bergner et al 1976a, Muldoon et al 1998). This tendency has since reversed, and instruments can be placed on a continuum from those that focus on measuring observable function (e.g. activities of daily living or ADL) to those that focus on patients' views of their condition or subjective well-being (e.g. see VanderZee et al 1996).

Some tests only assess factors that could be observed by an onlooker. A second group of tests are focused on patients' reports of how they feel or perceive their illness state, and are indifferent as to whether or not the report could be independently confirmed. A third group (such as those concerned with adaptation effects, see Ch. 2) actively seek a combination of the two.

Tests made up of elements that can be confirmed by an observer

There are situations where it is essential that the test is made up of elements that can be scored by an observer. These include:

- where patients are unable to communicate
- where gathering the information would be too burdensome for the patient
- where the patient is too young to provide assessments.

One important group is dying patients and their families. Steinhauser et al (2002) reviewed literature regarding QoL instruments used to assess the experiences of dying patients and concluded that because dying patients are often too ill to communicate, researchers must identify additional objective and subjective measures that can serve as valid alternatives to patients' self-ratings (see also Farsides & Dunlop 2001).

Children are often deemed to require proxy reports, although even relatively young children seem capable of independent report. Feeny et al (1998) assessed approaches for the assessment of HQoL in children with asthma, and concluded that children as young as 7 years may be able to reliably complete interviewer-administered, disease-specific and generic measures of HQoL, and by the age of 8 years, children seemed capable of completing a comprehensive battery of measures including direct preference measurement using a 'feeling thermometer'.

There are also situations where the patient could complete a measure, but where observer-based assessment is desirable. These include:

- where the report of the patient may be susceptible to bias (e.g. assessment for a pension)
- where the patient may lack the experience necessary to make an accurate estimate (e.g. whether requiring domiciliary or institutional care).

It has also been suggested that observer rating should be chosen as the principal outcome criterion in anti-depressant drug trials (e.g. Möller 2001).

Some hold the view that *all* assessments should only concern observables, a view more common in the past.

Thus Kaplan et al (1989) stated that 'most investigators believe that symptoms and mortality do represent quality of life' (Kaplan et al 1989, p. S31), contrasting this approach with those who regarded QoL as 'subjective appraisals of life satisfaction' (Hunt & McEwen 1983, cited in Kaplan et al 1989), or those who combine a patient's subjective evaluation of well-being with physical symptoms, sexual function, work performance, emotional status, etc. (Croog et al 1986, cited in Kaplan et al 1989).

In this respect, one might consider at least *two possible arguments* why QoL measures should be based exclusively on objective, externally observable attributes: 'non observables are banned', and 'only in development'.

'Non observables are banned'

A 'non observables are banned' position might state that any behaviour that cannot be directly observed is unworthy of measurement as it cannot be confirmed by an independent observer. This is the approach stated by Bergner et al (1976a) in the development of the SIP.

Such an approach makes determining the relative importance of different factors that might influence HQoL problematic, as is required in the common practice of assessing multiple dimensions and then combining them to form a global score. As the subject's own view of relative desirability would be precluded, one is left with seeking the views of 'experts' or arbitrarily assigning weightings to the dimensions/sub-scales.

Kaplan et al (1979) referred to this issue in advocating the rating of total case descriptions so that the effects of multiple dimensions of health could be estimated.

'Only in development'

A second position might state that any measure of HQoL reliant upon the report of an individual is liable to substantial measurement error, and it is preferable to develop an instrument that can be used to *predict* underlying HQoL independently of the subject's own report. Thus while subject report may be allowed a central role during instrument *development*, it is to be avoided in instrument application, i.e. when making a specific assessment.

Support for an approach that minimizes the role of a direct patient report of global HQoL also comes from evidence of adaptation/response bias, i.e. that direct report may be misleading (discussed in Ch. 2).

Finally, note that even for measures targeting factors that can theoretically be observed and confirmed by non-patients, the perception of the patient may be more valuable than that of an observer, as there is evidence that patient-rated symptoms have much better predictive value than clinician-rated ones (Chang et al 1998).

Tests measuring patient feelings and/or perceptions

While some may believe only observables should be included in tests, the more common approach is that HQoL tests need to assess health states as perceived by the patient.

For example, Gill & Feinstein (1994) argued that QoL was a uniquely personal perception denoting the way that individual patients feel about their health status and/or non-medical aspects of their lives, and that QoL can only be suitably measured by determining the opinions of patients. They also found that at that time, only 17% of HQoL measures allowed patients to give their own separate rating of QoL, and advocated supplementing (or replacing) instruments developed by 'experts'.

Consistent with this is the following definition of HQoL: 'Health-related quality of life refers to people's subjective evaluations of the influences of their current health status, healthcare, and health promoting activities on their ability to achieve and maintain a level of overall functioning that allows them to pursue valued life goals and that is reflected in their general well-being' (Shumaker et al 1997, p. 476).

Tests that embrace both objective and patient-subjective elements

Others have argued for the consideration of both objective and subjective information, particularly with HQoL in mental health conditions. Kastrup & Mezzich (2001) proposed that a central issue is the balance between subjective and objective judgement. On the other hand Muldoon et al (1998) observed that many QoL instruments produce composite indices that combine ratings of both functioning and subjective well-being, and argued that aggregating such disparate kinds of information was illogical.

The position taken here is that both types of variable have a potential place in a descriptive and predictive model of HQoL, as long as there are both theoretical and empirical grounds for selecting them. Using both patient-subjective and independently-observable variables may combat errors in one or the other and provide a comprehensive characterization of the condition.

Evidence of response-shift also argues for assessing observer-based as well as patient-reported measures, as discussed in Chapter 2.

FURTHER WAYS IN WHICH PATIENT-CENTRED MEASURES MAY BE DISTINGUISHED

The following outlines the major ways in which patient-centred measures may be distinguished, in addition to the subjective/objective dimension described above. Any one test may be distinguished in multiple ways, e.g. it may be based on subjective patient report, be disease-specific, etc.

Disease-specific versus generic measures

Some measures target a specific disease, others aspire to assess the effects of many or all forms of illness.

Disease-specific measures have greater salience for physicians, can focus on functional areas of particular concern, and may possess greater responsiveness to disease-specific interventions (Deyo & Patrick 1989, Patrick & Deyo 1989).

On the other hand, generic measures may in principle permit comparisons across interventions and diagnostic conditions, which is particularly important for policy makers. It also has been argued that generic measures can be as responsive in some settings as disease-specific measures: Kaplan et al (1989) criticized disease-specific methods on the grounds that all diseases and disabilities affect overall QoL, and the purpose of QoL measures is not to identify clinical information relevant to the disease but to determine the impact of the disease on general function.

Certainly a benefit of general measures is the ability to capture side effects and benefits that might not have been anticipated (Kaplan & Anderson 1988), however, a properly constructed disease-specific measure should be more capable of detecting slight changes in effects of particular interest. For example, Bennett et al (2002) compared two heart failure specific instruments and one generic instrument (the SF-12 [12-item short-form health survey], which is a subset of the SF-36; see Ware et al 1996) to measure HQoL in heart failure patients, and concluded that the disease-specific instruments were preferable. Also see Revicki et al (2000).

The issue may often be more apparent than real. Shumaker et al (1997) found that condition-specific instruments often contain both the broad, generic components of HQoL, as well as subscales or items specific to the symptoms and natural history associated with the condition and its treatment.

The pros and cons of generic tests

An emphasis on generic measures has been encouraged by the desire for standardization of instruments and the wish to assess across patient types and programmes. The SF-36 (Ware & Sherbourne 1992, McHorney et al 1993, Ware 1993) has been used to examine treatment effects across a broad range of illness conditions, including dialysis (Kurtin et al 1992), cardiac surgery (Phillips & Lansky 1992), and aged care (Weinberger et al 1991).

Almost by definition, generic instruments are not developed based on an intensive study or examination of illness-specific populations. There can be a problem when the instrument is applied to a specific group without intensively testing the capacity of the instrument against direct measurement of HQoL for that patient group (e.g. see Jayasuriya et al 1997). The desire to embrace generic tests is understandable, but of greater importance is that instruments measure what they are intended to. Instrument insensitivity could result in discrimination against effective treatments.

The problem is not just insensitivity but bias. The relative importance of dimensions of HQoL tend to differ according to the disease (Bernheim 1999) and to change with different stages of a disease (e.g. physical components become more important towards terminal stages: Chang et al 1998). Generic HQoL measures with a fixed scoring system may lead to some illness states being 'favoured' over others. Some illnesses are likely to be scored with considerable sensitivity, while for others the instruments may be relatively unresponsive.

No instrument can be assumed to be appropriate for the purpose without being evaluated. This issue is further discussed in Chapter 10.

The dimensions assessed

While by definition, disease-specific tests focus on the attributes/ dimensions most affected by the particular illness, generic tests also vary in the dimensions assessed. For example, Torrance (1987) considered that physiological and emotional functioning together constitute HQoL, but social functioning (e.g. social role and social contacts) lay outside the scope of HQoL. In contrast, Kaplan et al (1989) included social role, but did not include, e.g. the work setting.

Unfortunately an instrument may be applied to a particular group without considering whether the instrument assesses the domains of particular importance to the group. Carr & Higginson (2001) concluded that many generic tests fail to assess the QoL of patients through deficiencies in test structure and content, the ways in which they were developed, and their systems of domain weighting. For example, they found that patients with rheumatoid arthritis considered relationships and sexual functioning important, but these were not assessed by the SF-36, the EuroQoL, or the Nottingham health profile.

Similarly, Verkerk et al (2001) found that the SF-36 and the Nottingham health profile were unable to adequately assess the effect of introducing an integrated aged care system, as the questionnaires were judged unable to assess the important benefit of choice of access to activities. They concluded that standardized HQoL questionnaires failed when their functions or dimensions were not in line with the intervention being researched.

This issue is further discussed in Chapter 4 under 'Validity Evidence Based on Test Content'.

> **The range of dimensions sampled when estimating HQoL is central to the validity of HQoL measures. Which dimensions to include should depend on the purpose of the test.**

Tests that provide only a 'profile' and not an overall score

The Medical Outcomes Study (MOS) 36-item short-form health survey (or SF-36; Ware & Sherbourne 1992) is often described as providing only a 'profile' of scores, i.e. a set of sub-scale measures, emphasizing the value of explicitly assessing and reporting a number of important dimensions of HQoL. In contrast, the Quality of Well-Being index (Kaplan et al 1976) provides a single score estimate to assist resource allocation decisions.

There is no reason why a test cannot both provide an overall estimate of HQoL and a breakdown of values per dimension, and most do. (In fact the SF-36 does provide an overall measure with its first item: 'In general, would you say your health is: Excellent Very Good   Good   Fair   Poor'.)

Tests aiming to measure 'utility'

Many tests have been developed to assist the rational allocation of healthcare resources. For example, it is argued that rational allocation should be based on evaluating the benefits of medical care expressed in terms of output in years of life adjusted by the QoL of those years (Kaplan & Anderson 1988, Kaplan et al 1989).

In health economics, the measures of QoL used are described as 'utility' measures, with 'utility' traditionally equated with 'strength of preference', in the sense that state A has greater 'utility' than state B if state A is preferred to state B. Measures of the utility of health states may then be input to cost-utility analysis (CUA), a form of cost-effectiveness analysis, that 'focuses on the quality of health outcome caused or averted by health programs or treatments' (Drummond et al 1987, p. 112).

CUA measures health improvement in units such as quality adjusted life years (QALYs), which aim simultaneously to incorporate quantity of life (years left to live) with QoL (the value of each year lived). The quality adjustment is based on the measurement of the utilities for each possible health state, reflecting the relative desirability of the health state: an increase in life of 10 years where each year has a utility value of 0.5 would represent a gain of 5 QALYs (10 × 0.5).

Note that the boundaries of what is referred to as utility are currently expanding and becoming fused with more general notions of the degree to which health states are viewed and experienced as desirable/undesirable (see Kahneman 2000, and the following chapter).

Utility measures are considered further in Chapter 11 under 'Measuring Utilities'.

Tests measuring patient perceptions of healthcare

Patient satisfaction may be defined as patients' (or their families') emotional or cognitive evaluation of a healthcare experience. Kane (1997) suggested that reasons for measuring satisfaction included:

- Patients can play an important role in defining how healthcare is delivered.
- Patients can play an important role in defining quality of care by determining what values should be associated with different outcomes.
- Physicians' interpersonal skills influence patient outcomes.
- Satisfaction can improve outcomes through a placebo effect.
- Medical care was becoming more a consumer good so patient satisfaction was more salient.

The measurement of patient satisfaction entails similar issues to generic and specific health status measurement. There is often a tradeoff between coverage and depth; a clear definition of why/ what to measure is essential, and both a global measure and a sub-scale structure is desirable. Sub-scale scores allow the instrument to play a diagnostic role and identify the relative importance of different dimensions in determining satisfaction.

Ware et al (1978) provided an early review of the area, while McKinley et al (1997), Ryan & Farrar (2000), and Gardner & Chapple (1999) authored more recent reports. See Bond & Fox (2001, p. 142) for the application of Rasch modelling to satisfaction data.

Tests measuring impact on families

Families often provide continuing care for a chronically ill relative, whether through choice or necessity, and the measurement of family burden has become an increasing focus of tests.

Again, the same issues apply as in measuring HQoL, i.e. identifying objective and subjective dimensions of family burden, and the extent to which illness characteristics and other variables contribute to care giver stress for different chronic illnesses (e.g. Sales 2003).

Measuring family satisfaction with healthcare given to the patient may also be assessed (e.g. Ringdal et al 2003).

Tests that aim to model behaviour and predict avoidable events

Most tests characterize a passive state that may in part result from undesirable health-related behaviours. However, there is considerable potential for tests that are able to identify the behaviours themselves, and potentially predict events that could be avoided if there is a suitable intervention.

An example of such a test is the Asthma Medication Adherence Questionnaire (AMAQ), based on estimates of factors such as relationship with the doctor and non-adherent behaviours (O'Connor et al 2000). These issues are discussed more fully under 'Dynamic Measures' in Chapter 11.

SUMMARY

- Factors responsible for the development of patient-centred measures are:
  - The need to assess the relative merits of health programmes

  – The desire to comprehensively assess the impact of clinical therapies
  – The recognition that patients have a different view of their health from their doctors
  – The potential benefits for clinical practice.
- Patient-centred health outcome measures are measures that aim to assess and promote health (and healthcare) as it is perceived and experienced by patients. Measures of HQoL are the most numerous members of this group.
- For HQoL/health status measures, there is no common reporting method and a wide variation in terminology; much of the terminology is also interchangeable. Hence it is essential to determine how terms are *actually being used* in health outcome measurement studies, particularly the phrase 'quality of life'. Readers should always conduct their own assessment of the degree to which such measures include relevant dimensions, are based on patient report, etc.
- The classes of test and/or ways in which patient-centred measures differ include:
  – Tests requiring subjective patient report versus tests based on observables
  – Tests made up of elements that can be confirmed by an observer
  – Tests measuring patient feelings and/or perceptions
  – Tests that embrace both objective and patient-subjective elements
  – Disease-specific versus generic measures
  – The dimensions assessed
  – Tests that provide only a 'profile' and not an overall score
  – Tests providing a 'utility'
  – Tests measuring quality of healthcare
  – Tests measuring family burden
  – Tests that aim to model behaviour and predict avoidable events.

KEY ISSUES ADDRESSED IN THIS BOOK

Which is the right test?
Healthcare workers frequently feel unsure as to which test, if any, is suitable for their population. Bottomley (2002) reviewed surveys on

the views of oncologists, and found that while most believed that HQoL information should be collected from patients, there was confusion about the measure to use and the adequacy of current measurement tools.

Chapters 3, 4, and 5 set out issues to be considered when selecting or developing a test, and Chapter 10 provides a test evaluation template.

How was the test created? How was it constructed?
Classical Test Theory and its summed-scale approach are fairly easy to understand. In contrast, Modern Test Theory, i.e. models associated with Item Response Theory and the Rasch model, requires a considerably higher degree of effort and explanation.

Chapters 6 and 7 describe test development under Classical Test Theory, and Chapter 8 describes the nature of Item Response Theory/Rasch theory and issues in developing a test based on the Rasch model.

What do the results mean? How are they interpreted? How might a test be used in a clinical as opposed to research setting?
Improved ways of analyzing, applying, presenting and understanding test results are very important both for developing more valid tests and interpreting the results. A new and critical issue is how to deal with the recognition that patients play a dynamic role in experiencing, perceiving, and assessing their HQoL. HQoL tests also need to be interpretable in clinical terms if they are to enter fully into clinical practice.

These issues are discussed in a number of chapters and sections from varying vantage points, including Chapters 2, 8, and 11 under 'Interpreting Quality of Life Scores for Individual Patients'.

2

Diverse psychological mechanisms mediate reports of health-related quality of life

---

AIMS OF CHAPTER

- To reveal the broad range of psychological mechanisms that are likely to influence patient perception and report

- To demonstrate that simple additive models may not accurately indicate health-related quality of life as perceived by patients

---

There is an extensive and growing body of literature spread across several research areas (including utility measurement, subjective well-being, and quality of life [QoL]/health-related quality of life [HQoL]) revealing that diverse psychological mechanisms mediate people's reports regarding health states.

People are active participants in their own states. Psychological processes influence the perception and report of HQoL, whether by the patient or another. This chapter describes how people actively participate in the perception, emoting, appraisal, and recall of situations and experiences.

PATIENT DECISION-MAKING HAS SEEMINGLY NON-RATIONAL FEATURES

Patients do not gather all available information about their situation, calculate the costs and benefits of alternatives, and then make the optimal choice. People seem to use short-hand decision methods that can lead to sub-optimal decisions. As described by Redelmeier et al (1993), these include:

Loss aversion

People take losses far more seriously than foregone gains, hence they are reluctant to accept a loss in one dimension of life to achieve an improvement in another. (This implies that time-tradeoff tasks are inherently questionable; see Saigal et al 2001.)

A poor ability to predict future feelings or preferences

Predictions about future actions are inaccurate; people change their minds when they confront a particular situation.

Referring to the 'hot/cold empathy gap', Loewenstein & Schkade (1997) gave as examples: the majority of women reverse their decision not to use anaesthesia in childbirth once actually in labour (even those who had previously had children); current cancer patients accept grueling chemotherapy when healthy people say they would not; and dying patients accept heroic care in acute hospitals when healthy people say they wish to die at home.

The clear evidence is that non-patients, or patients not undergoing a particular condition, are not good judges. This feature undermines the arguments of some health economists that the general public should provide the judgements of the 'utility' of health states (given decisions are different when the health state is entered).

Memories are inaccurate representations of experiences

Memories of events can be inaccurate. For example, the same amount of severe pain is less aversive in retrospect if immediately followed by moderate pain, as recalled affect is determined by the worst state and the end-state, not a sum of all states, e.g. see Redelmeier & Kahneman 1996. In other words, an experience may be bad when being experienced but okay in retrospect, encouraging choice of a treatment that was more unpleasant when experienced but that has been remembered more favourably.

'Framing' effects

People's decisions depend on both the experience referred to and the way in which it is presented or 'framed'.

People tend to be unaware of the extent to which preferences can be altered by a subtle change in formulation. For example, patients are likely to respond differently if informed that 'there is a 10% mortality following the procedure' as opposed to 'there is 90% survival'. This indicates considerable care is needed when phrasing questions, clinically or in a test (all test instructions should be standardized and rely minimally on instructions from test presenters, trained or otherwise).

Irrational concerns

An irrational concern is, e.g. the 'law of contagion', which is an unwillingness to have contact with objects, even when sterilized, that have been in contact with a person or thing that was ill or infected (Rozin & Nemeroff 1990).

Inability to control worries

There is often inability to control worries, even where this may be counterproductive. An example is avoidance of cancer screening.

DISPOSITIONAL SUBJECTIVE WELL-BEING MAY INFLUENCE REPORT

Subjective well-being (SWB), is generally treated as consisting of life satisfaction and the presence of positive mood and the absence of negative mood (Ryan & Deci 2001).

A number of researchers have phrased HQoL in terms of subjective well-being. Donovan et al (1989) suggested that an accepted general definition of QoL is 'a person's subjective sense of well-being, derived from current experience of life as a whole'. In the context of treatment selection, Goodinson & Singleton (1989) propose a definition of QoL as 'the degree of satisfaction with perceived present life circumstances', this being seen to encompass the 'physical, social, and material well-being of an individual', and to concern an evaluation of the physical, psychological and social impact of disease treatment on patients' lives.

People are generally happy but differ in characteristic levels of happiness

Research into subjective well-being indicates that people seem to feel some affect during virtually all of their waking moments, and all affect seems to be either pleasant or unpleasant. In fact, most people report having positive affect most of the time (Diener & Lucas 2000).

SWB also has trait-like features, distinguishing one individual from another. Some people seem chronically happy and others chronically unhappy. Happy people tend to interpret the same life events more favourably than unhappy people, casting the life events in a more positive light, because they are less responsive to negative feedback, and more strongly denigrate opportunities not available to them (Ryan & Deci 2001). People seem to be predisposed to experience certain emotions, and personality factors may contribute to the creation of life circumstances that foster pleasant or unpleasant emotional experiences (Diener & Lucas 2000). Personality traits are highly stable and may predict SWB 20 years later (cf. Heady & Wearing 1989).

Positive affect seems to be associated with better health

An emphasis on positive events may be the norm rather than the exception and may lead to a longer life. A study of the diaries of Catholic nuns found that positive emotions experienced early in life predicted longevity more than 60 years later (Walker et al 2003, citing Danner et al 2001). A possible mechanism for positive affect being associated with better health was identified by Rosenkranz et al (2003), who found that individuals characterized by more negative affect produced a weaker immune response.

It has been suggested that optimism might be cultivated to facilitate SWB and improved health. Yu et al (2003) suggested the possible benefit of cultivating optimism to aid adaptation and recovery. Investigating eating difficulties after radiotherapy for nasopharyngeal carcinoma, Yu et al concluded that optimism significantly assisted eating ability and overall HQoL and argued that facilitating positive thinking may assist post-radiation adjustment. (See also Wrosch & Scheier 2003, Schneiderman et al 2001.)

There are slight effects of mood on reported well-being and more substantial cultural effects

It seems reasonable to expect that transient mood affects will influence reported well-being (Yardley & Rice 1991, Croyle & Uretsky 1987); however, Diener & Lucas (2000) concluded that the effect seemed small. On the other hand, there are a range of reports suggesting that cultures differ in the degree to which well-being is influenced by environmental variables or are sustained by personality characteristics (see Ch. 11, under 'Cross-cultural Application Issues').

HUMANS ADAPT TO ADVERSE HEALTH STATES

There are a broad range of results suggesting the presence of general psychological mechanisms that act to increase reported SWB (e.g. see Breetvelt & Van Dam 1991). Adaptation can be so great as to apparently eliminate SWB differences between chronically ill people and controls or even those who have recently had very positive experiences. For example, Brickman et al (1978) reported that lottery winners and quadriplegics differed little from normal controls in SWB. Similarly, Waldron et al (1999) examined patients with advanced incurable cancer and concluded that many rated their QoL as good.

Note that the relationship between health and SWB may be bi-directional. Hughes (1985) found that depression following lung cancer radiotherapy may exacerbate symptom distress (tiredness, anorexia, pain). Donovan et al (1989) also pointed out that cancer patients experience positive impacts of the disease on their life as well as negative, e.g. increased closeness to spouse.

Deteriorating states 'adapt' more than improving ones

Positive affect may also exhibit adaptation, for example marriage (see Lucas et al 2003). However, adaptation seems to apply more to negative affect. Walker et al (2003) reviewed a range of evidence and concluded that most people perceive their lives to be more positive than negative, and that negative emotions associated with bad events tend to diminish while positive emotions associated with good events tend to persist.

Adaptation may also be greater in deteriorating states than improving ones, as indicated by a study that compared retrospective reports with evidence gathered at the time. Cella et al (2002b) assessed cancer patients with the Functional Assessment of Cancer Therapy (FACT), and then later gathered retrospective global ratings of change. They found that the relationship between actual change scores and retrospective ratings was modest but usually statistically significant. However, those who reported global worsening had considerably larger change scores than those reporting comparable global improvements. In other words, small gains in HRQL had substantial value for patients, while comparable declines seemed less meaningful. Patients seemed to minimize declines and exaggerate improvements.

> **Adaptation works to minimize the impact of adverse states. If a test based on subject patient-report indicates that HQoL has deteriorated, it probably has.**

ADAPTATION MAY INCLUDE A RE-SETTING OF EXPECTATIONS

A major determinant of an individual's subjective QoL may be the perceived discrepancy between what is and what could have been (cf. Calman 1984, Skeel 1989). Well-being may be a function of expecting to attain, and ultimately attaining, the outcomes one values (Ryan & Deci 2001).

Campbell (1981) reported that when questioned about the quality of their lives, apparently healthy individuals respond in terms of life satisfaction, usually in relation to specific domains where satisfaction is proportional to the closeness between aspiration and achievement. Bergner (1989) also reports the notion that QoL is enhanced as the distance between attained and desired goals diminishes.

As expressed by Carr et al (2001), existing measures of QoL do not account for expectations of health. Someone with an experience of poor health who has low expectations might not evaluate a given

experience as having an impact on their QoL because their expectations are correspondingly low; conversely someone with good
health might report a significant impact on their QoL from a relatively minor illness, such as tonsillitis, because they have high
expectations of their health.

In this vein, it has been suggested that adaptation entails the
re-setting of aspirations or expectations, and/or a change in reference standards, leading to improved well-being/QoL. This may
also be referred to as 'response shift' – the idea that the terms of
reference by which QoL is judged change over time.

Adaptation is normally highly effective but may be incomplete
when objective conditions are particularly poor

Despite adaptation, SWB is influenced by life events and experiences (Diener 1984, Heady et al 1985, Heady & Wearing 1989,
Diener et al 1999); this includes the effects of poor health. However,
adaptation may fail with particularly undesirable experiences.

Cummins (2000) reviewed empirical data regarding the relationship between objective and subjective QoL indicators, including health conditions. He argued that subjective QoL (e.g. as
expressed in life satisfaction) is normally maintained within a
narrow range despite variation in objective factors (such as functional status), so objective and subjective indicators are normally
poorly correlated; however, very poor objective conditions can
defeat homeostasis, so objective and subjective indicators then
display a stronger relationship. Consistent with this, Diener &
Diener (1995) found that financial status was more correlated
with life satisfaction in poorer nations than wealthier nations,
while Watten et al (1997) found little relationship between SWB
and health in army recruits. See also Fakhoury & Priebe (2002).

THE COMPLEX INTERPLAY BETWEEN
EXPERIENCE, AFFECT AND COGNITIVE
EVALUATION

Are they happy or do they just say they are? (or
'satisfied with life' and unhappy at the same time)

There is an unhelpful fusion in the general literature on SWB
covering both affective and cognitive reactions (Diener et al 1999
provide a contemporary review of the area). As noted, subjective

well-being can refer to emotional factors, i.e. feeling happy/ unhappy, and/or cognitive factors where subjects are questioned regarding life satisfaction ('are you satisfied with your life?').

This leads to confusion and a need for considerable caution, as patients can respond differently depending upon which of the two notions of SWB they are asked to report on. For example, in comparing cancer patients with healthy persons, VanderZee et al (1996) found that psychological stress expressed as a depressed state was significantly greater in cancer patients. Nonetheless, it was argued that 'subjective well-being' was not affected, as life satisfaction measures did not differ.

It is important to recognize that the term SWB can be ambiguous, and to clearly distinguish whether positive affect (emotional state of 'happiness') or a cognitive appraisal of global life circumstances (judged 'satisfaction') is being investigated: if patients are asked about 'life satisfaction', then little difference may be found between patients and healthy persons; if 'happiness' is measured, then patients may be found to have less SWB.

There is other evidence that patient report of SWB is not always that convincing, e.g. it may conflict with the views of carers.

Epstein et al (1989) asked family/friend care givers to act as proxies for older chronically ill patients. It was found that while proxy and patient responses were similar for overall health, functional status, and social activity, proxies rated subjects' emotional health and satisfaction significantly lower than did the subjects themselves.

Kahneman (2000) suggested that studies of 'treadmill' effects (i.e. return to some pre-set level of happiness) are not entirely persuasive, and that it is a cognitive process that is responsible, not a change in actual happiness.

If patients make judgements relative to an internal criterion that is in some way adjusted to bring about a positive report, then cognitive factors may lead to 'under reporting', i.e. that 'patients report less emotional distress, satisfaction or the like than is actually present' (Breetvelt & Van Dam 1991, p. 983).

There is evidence that such under-reporting may diminish as distance in time from the unpleasant state increases. Thus Adang et al (1998) found that kidney transplant patients gave increasingly *negative* retrospective estimates of the HQoL they had pre-transplant as distance in time increased from when transplantation took place: the longer the time since the transplant, the worse they reported pre-transplant HQoL had been.

> When asking about SWB, recognize that questions
> regarding affect (Are you feeling happy?) and questions
> regarding satisfaction (How satisfied are you?) probably
> measure different things.

Reported affect does not accurately reflect experience(s): the 'peak/end' rule

There is other evidence that patient report may understate the negative value of experience.

In what will doubtless become a classic experiment, Redelmeier & Kahneman (1996) studied reports of pain during colonoscopies. Measures were taken of pain intensity in real-time pain by patients' recording experiences every 60 seconds using a visual analogue scale (VAS) (ends denoted 'no pain' and 'extreme pain').

In addition, patients' memories of the total amount of pain experienced were gathered with judgements of the 'total amount of pain experienced' (within 1 hour and 1 month after the procedure). The attending physician was also asked (immediately after the procedure) to estimate how the patient would subsequently rate the total amount of pain experienced.

The results indicated no apparent relationship between the duration of a procedure and the patients' subsequent evaluation of it ($r = 0.03$). However, the patients' subsequent evaluation of the procedure was able to be predicted based on a combination of the most intense level of pain reported during the procedure and the mean pain level reported over the last 3 minutes ($r = 0.67$), known as the 'peak/end rule'. The physicians report also correlated highly with the patients retrospective report ($r = 0.67$).

Other research has indicated that even when the sum of pain intensities is the same, the increasing pain intensity is perceived as very painful, and decreasing intensity as not painful (Ariely 1998).

Diener & Lucas (2000) also reported the finding that judgements of well-being do not seem to be based on simple aggregations of the amount of pleasant affect.

Much further work is needed to tease out the way that frequency and intensity of experiences influence retrospective judgements of affect.

Kahneman's nomenclature for considering the subjective well-being/'utility' of a state

The results that have been described suggest that considerable care is needed when generalizing about the HQoL of a health state. As stated by Diener & Lucas (2000) in the context of subjective emotional well-being, the type of response scale that is used, the response options, and the order and presentation of questions, can all influence the levels of HQoL that individuals report (citing Schwarz & Strack 1991).

In an attempt to categorize findings and clarify thinking, given the evidence that different answers emerge depending on if an individual is asked about an anticipated state, a current state, or a recalled state, Kahneman (2000) proposed four distinct classes of 'utility of outcome'.

This typology was seen to encompass evidence from decision studies and SWB/QoL findings. 'Utility' in this context referred to a general notion of judged and/or experienced desirability/undesirability of a state. Four classes of utility were proposed: decision, predicted, moment-based, and remembered.

1. 'Decision utility'

Decision utility refers to utility as inferred from observed preferences, described as the almost exclusive topic of study in decision research and economics.

2. 'Predicted utility'

This refers to beliefs concerning future health states. As described earlier in this chapter, people's decisions and preferences tend to change when they find themselves actually in the situation (the 'hot/cold empathy gap'; Loewenstein & Schkade 1997).

3. 'Total utility', 'moment-based utility' or 'experienced utility'

This measure is based on measures of real-time pleasure/pain (Redelmeier & Kahneman 1996).

Kahneman (2000) argues that memory-based measures 'may not tell us what we really want to know'. Thus while 'people who move to California' seem to report no more happiness than those in seemingly less desirable locations, Kahneman argues that they may actually be found to be happier *if they are assessed by moment-based measures.*

Kahneman argues that moment-based utility corresponds to objective happiness, and that experienced utility and objective happiness may be the correct measure of welfare for comparisons of groups (e.g. Californians and others) or assessments of the value of public goods such as health insurance.

4. 'Remembered utility' – retrospective assessments of episodes or periods of life

As described by Kahneman, remembered utility is the almost exclusive topic of study in SWB research.

As found by the colonoscopies studied by Redelmeier & Kahneman (1996), recalled pain was a transformed function of experienced pain (the peak/end rule). Questions regarding 'satisfaction with life' also seem to exhibit a transformation of the experience, although of a different type.

A survival perspective of 'adaptation and augmentation'?

The following speculates on the possible functions indicated by the phenomena discussed.

There is evidence that adaptation is dynamic in the sense that states are re-appraised to allow severely adverse affect to be consciously recognized when it is 'safe' to do so (cf. Adang et al 1998).

The peak/end rule (Redelmeier & Kahneman 1996) suggests that improving states are viewed more tolerantly, i.e. with less negative affect, than deteriorating ones, even where the total amount of pain is the same. This seems to be a response that could have survival benefits, given improving states would tend to be less hazardous than deteriorating ones.

Perhaps there is a general principle of dynamic adaptation/augmentation, such that:

- successive improving states or 'changes for the better' are found rewarding, pursued, and perhaps enhanced or augmented, but then (to some extent) diminished when past

• deteriorating states or 'changes for the worse' are found
  punishing/hazardous, retreated from, and adapted to the
  extent necessary to maintain optimal functioning without
  ignoring the lesson.

Indeed if euphoria and depression did not return to an early
moderate state, people would be immune to reward or punish-
ment and possibly lose their capacity to adapt to a changing environment. A state of mild positive affect and optimism (associated
with positive action?) is one that meets this requirement, and is
seemingly the most common.

Furthermore the two aspects of SWB (rational consideration of
current state as indicated when replying to questions regarding
'satisfaction with life', and degree of affect), may signal underlying complementary functions: affect provides a necessary, immediate indication of pleasure/pain, and hence benefit/hazard,
spurring action to be taken when needed. At the same time the
negative value of past affect is regulated and limited, as reflected
in 'judged satisfaction'.

THE GLOBAL EVALUATION OF AN EXPERIENCED STATE IS NOT THE SUM OF ITS PARTS

A primary lesson to draw from the information in this chapter is
that reflective or retrospective evaluations of experienced health
states are mediated by a complex range of psychological processes
that represent anything but a simple summation of experience.

This is evident in the 'peak/end rule' of Redelmeier & Kahneman
(1996) with selective recall of a past health state seeming to occur
almost immediately, and patient reports exhibiting an abstracted
and transformed version of experience. More generally, there seems
to be a principle whereby people systematically act to discount the
impact of selected experiences and to possibly augment others, as
indicated, e.g. by the report of Cella et al (2002b) in which cancer
patients seemed to minimize declines and exaggerate improvements when giving retrospective ratings of change in HQoL.

There is other evidence to support the notion that reported (perceived?) QoL is not the sum or average of experience, but represents
a general function of the selective discounting of adverse experiences. For example, Redelmeier & Kahneman (1996) found that, as
well as the patients, attending physicians predicted the amount of

pain experienced by the patients during colonoscopy suggesting that they, too, applied the 'peak/end rule', emphasizing the most severe experience instead of summing up all negative experiences.

A similar result was reported by Bergner et al (1976a) when developing a scoring mechanism for the Sickness Impact Profile (SIP). They found that in developing global estimates of dysfunction, the judges appeared to attend to both the number of items checked and the items checked with the highest values, not the mean score across all items. Similar results were found by O'Connor et al (1996) when developing a measure of work-related disability: the best predictor of the global assessment of a given patient by medical officers was found to be the score of the highest-rated disability of the patient, not the total of all disabilities.

Perhaps a further illustration of this principle was given by Primo Levi in *If This Is A Man* (Levi 1987), an account of his experiences in a concentration camp. Levi explained how he thought only of the most pressing need at a time (e.g. reaching the head of the meal queue), and that if he had considered all of the problems he faced he could not have coped. By concentrating only on the most pressing need, he survived.

Overall evaluations of experienced health states are not the sum or average.

The reported value of a negative health state experience formed of multiple elements is best predicted by the most affecting aspect of the experience.
  The best rule for predicting affect/HQoL may be a combination of salience and spread, or the end versus preceding, improving versus deteriorating, etc. It is unlikely to be a simple addition of the values of the individual elements.

FURTHER IMPLICATIONS: INCLUDE OBSERVABLE VARIABLES AS WELL AS SUBJECTIVE PATIENT REPORT

HQoL can be assessed by objective (e.g. functional status measures) and subjective indicators (reports of SWB). Given the substantial but unclear affects of adaptation, multiple means of assessing HQoL seem desirable.

Diener & Lucas (2000) also recommended that multiple methods be used when estimating a person's subjective emotional well-being, including peer (or carer) reports and non-verbal behaviours. They argued that methods beyond the subjects' own reports were essential, and that when all measures converged, one could have greater confidence in the results.

SUMMARY

Reports of HQoL are influenced by factors other than external events or physical conditions. Considered self-reports of HQoL may also differ from affective HQoL, i.e. they may suggest a more positive state than the patient is actually experiencing (a patient's report may indicate a 'coming to terms'; it does not mean that they would not greatly prefer an alternative state).

Current measures are generally not designed to distinguish between changes in the experience of disease and changes in expectations of health or reports of health (Carr et al 2001), and adaptation/response shifts may need to be tracked and quantified for a proper interpretation of subjective QoL results in 'before-after' designs (Bar-On et al 2000). See also Stiggelbout & de Haes (2001) and Norman (2003).

There is a need to attempt to measure variables relevant to adaptation. For example, illnesses may differ in the extent to which they allow adaptation.

Illnesses where acuity fluctuates, or is uncertain, may be less readily adapted to, compared to stable conditions where the prognosis is clear.

A growing range of issues need research, which include:

- the factors and conditions determining the rate and extent of adaptation/augmentation
- whether both satisfaction and affect adapt in the same way (the evidence suggests they may not)
- the relative contributions of satisfaction and affect to adaptation generally
- the relationship between affect and appraisal
- the relative value of memories versus experiences
- whether healthcare workers also experience adaptation (this may explain the diminishing relationship between

patient report and doctor as doctors become more experienced)
- the degree to which patients 'ignore' unpalatable information to assist their adaptation, and the complex issues relating to 'deception' by healthcare personnel (e.g. see Sade 2001)
- whether adaptation aids recovery, perhaps via the production of positive affect
- whether adaptation plays a role in the placebo effect
- ways to ask questions of patients that may tease out these issues and possible ethical issues if such questioning leads to a reduction in adaptation.

KEY POINTS

- Psychological mechanisms influence patient reports of HQoL, and psychological processes operate to increase SWB/QoL.
- Different answers are likely to be obtained depending on whether inquiry is made regarding an anticipated, current, or recalled health state.
- Self-reported QoL may suggest a more positive state than the patient is actually experiencing, particularly if asking for a cognitive appraisal (e.g. satisfaction with life) as opposed to a report of current affect (are you feeling happy right now?).
- Where possible, assess *both* affect (happiness/unhappiness) as well as the patient's cognitive appraisal (i.e. 'all things considered' questions).
- Global reports may not give an accurate indication of the real-time experience of the situation.
- Rules for estimating the HQoL of complex states are unlikely to be a simple addition of the parts.
- There is a value in multiple measures, including objective as well as subjective indicators, and carer report as well as patient report.
- Finally, adaptation seems to work to minimize the impact of adverse states. If a test based on subjective patient-report indicates that HQoL has deteriorated, it probably has.

3

First actions when selecting, assessing, developing or modifying a test

---

AIMS OF CHAPTER

- To indicate the first actions to be taken before selecting a test or developing a new test

- To stress the importance of being absolutely clear on what the user's needs are and that these need to be defined and specified in as much detail as possible

---

Health outcome tests will only provide the necessary information if the healthcare agency using the test is clear on its own needs and the role of the test in supporting those needs.

SPECIFY THE PURPOSE TO WHICH THE TEST WILL BE PUT AND THE CONCEPT TO BE USED

What is the purpose of the test as defined by the test user?

This question is the first question to be answered when selecting, assessing, developing or modifying a health outcomes test and it must be answered. It is fundamental to assessment of the test's validity, which in essence is 'the ability of the test to measure what it is intended to measure'. Obviously, if it is not clear what the test is intended to achieve, it is very difficult to confirm whether or not the test can achieve its purpose!

One way of considering this question is to determine the practical decision that needs to be made (explicitly or by default) and that the test is intended to help with. The test may be intended to aid decisions regarding the effectiveness of treatment for individual patients. Alternatively, it may be required to assess the effectiveness of a hospital programme or a state-wide programme.

It is usually difficult (it can be *very* difficult) to specify the purpose of the test. The reason is that programmes often operate for historical reasons, and if the purpose of the healthcare programme or treatment is unclear, then the purpose of any test that aims to assess an element of that programme is also likely to be unclear. Such specification of purpose is necessary to ensure that the instrument is capable of performing the task demanded of it.

What is the attribute/ability to be measured?

This question is the second question to be answered and indicates that the next issue is to resolve the construct (attribute/ability) to be measured. For example, the purpose of the test may be 'to determine if the treatment is effective and should be continued'. Such a purpose does not specify what is to be measured to make the decision. There are a range of constructs that could be measured, e.g.:

- ability to carry out the activities of daily living
- health-related quality of life (HQoL) as globally assessed by the patient
- ability to return to work
- medication adherence
- extent of self-injurious behaviour, etc.

One way of considering this is to determine what the test is to help maximize. The attribute/construct that is to be measured and what it is desired to maximize needs to be explored and defined.

The two questions above can be, and need to be, clearly and unambiguously resolved. Both the selector/developer of the measurement instrument and the users of the instrument then know what the job of the test is, can determine how well it does it, and can also begin to determine how well the programme is doing in the achievement of its purpose.

This process can lead to the application of a valid and effective instrument, and help the programme itself become more efficient and effective.

Where applicable, specify a criterion/ proxy-criterion

There has been a disregard of criterion measures in theoretical accounts of the development of patient-centred health outcome measures, when almost by definition, patients' own assessments of their conditions are generally available as candidates (where the test is one based on observable variables, an 'expert's' view may at times be preferred).

Criterion measures in HQoL measurement are discussed in considerable detail in Chapter 5 under 'Global ratings as Criterion Measures in Test Development' and in Chapter 4 under 'Criterion-related validity'.

In the meantime, it is useful to conceive of the purpose, construct, and criterion as successive efforts to make the task of the test more focused and concrete. The criterion represents an operationalization of the construct. Where the operationalization is considered a rough approximation, the term 'proxy-criterion' may be preferred. For examples, see Box 3.1.

Box 3.1   Examples of purpose, construct, and proxy-criterion

Example 1: Development of work ability tables (O'Connor et al 1996)

Purpose: Assess the degree of work-related disability to assist allocation of pensions.

Construct: 'Work-related disability'.

Proxy-criterion: Assessment by medical officers regarding an applicant's ability to work using a 0–100 visual analogue scale (VAS), with 0 labelled 'no reduction in ability to work' and 100 'totally unable to work'. Note that the judgement of applicants could be considered biased due to self interest in being judged unable to work.

Example 2: Development of Asthma Medication Adherence Questionnaire or AMAQ (funded by Glaxo SmithKline; O'Connor et al 2000)

Purpose: Estimate adherence to asthma preventer medication based on patient-reported attitudes and behaviours.

Construct: Degree to which patient took medication as directed by doctor.

Proxy-criterion: Patient's confidential report of preventer medication use over the 24 hours prior to measurement.

The more focused the task, the easier it is to develop a valid tool. In the experience of the author, when the instrument has been developed to aid a specific health programme decision, there is almost always a proxy-criterion against which the instrument can be assessed.

IDENTIFY CRITERIA THE TEST NEEDS TO MEET

Having determined the purpose of the test and the construct to be measured, the aspects of the test that will determine its effectiveness need to be considered and written down. These aspects form the criteria the test needs to meet.

To the extent that such criteria are *not* considered, the process of developing/selecting the test will be confused and undergo setbacks, as required features are progressively identified and found absent. The more criteria are specified at the beginning, the less wasted effort will occur later. In the worse case, a test could be introduced for use and then found unsuitable.

Criteria should concern practical in-use features of the test such as time to administer and whether or not it provides an overall score, elements of the test development process (e.g. who is/was consulted in identifying content), and the degree to which the test meets conditions of validity, reliability and scaling. In support of such an approach, Shumaker et al (1997) discussed the assessment of instruments for measuring human immunodeficiency virus (HIV) HQoL. They proposed that criteria should be developed and applied to each candidate test, with the instruments then 'scored' by the degree to which they met each criterion. This was seen to help identify current shortcomings as well as locate instruments holding the most promise of moving the field forward.

The following discusses the types of criteria it is worthwhile to consider. Criteria should be detailed as far as possible, but should include at least the 'practical needs criteria'.

Practical needs criteria

Size and time to complete

Measurement tasks need to be readily understood and administered in a reasonable time (Donovan et al 1989), both from the point of view of the patient, and demands placed on staff resources.

Shorter tests may be needed by older or disabled persons (Deyo & Patrick 1989). The item type is also relevant. Questions with a limited number of fixed alternatives are likely to be quicker to complete than an instrument employing continuous or visual analogue scales (VASs) (Donovan et al 1989).

While brevity and simplicity are important so that the test can achieve its purpose, longer tests can be more reliable and valid (although Modern Test Theory is capable of making shorter tests of equal validity; see Chs 6 and 8). On the other hand, even single item tests can play a valuable role if they are carefully constructed (see Ch. 5 under 'The Role of Patient Global Self-ratings').

Interviewer-administered versus self-administered tests

A decision needs to be made between interviewer-administered and self-administered tests. Interviewer-administered tests might reduce the burden on patients (Revicki 1989), but can place greater demands on staff resources and might be less reliable.

Tests requiring the items to be asked of the patient/client should require trained interviewers. In practice, there is often great variation in the extent to which such training has been received, and the administrators may have had no special training at all. This introduces additional undesirable error variance into the results.

Even when training has been received, it may be of limited effectiveness. Lumley & McNamara (1995) examined the training of raters for the speaking subtest of the Occupational English Test (OET) for health professionals who intend to practice in Australia. They found substantial variation in tester estimates that training was unable to eliminate or reduce to acceptable levels, and the effects of training often diminished rapidly.

The mode of administration also affects the results received. Evidence suggests that interviewer delivery of a test is valuable, but it is then best that the patient completes the test alone. Bergner et al (1981) examined three types of administration:

- administration by interviewer
- delivery and explanation by interviewer, and then self-administration
- delivery by mail and self-administration.

Bergner et al (1981) concluded that delivery by interviewer and self-administration was the best, producing the highest correlations between Sickness Impact Profile (SIP) scores and self-assessed dysfunction and illness. Interviewer administration was the next best. The worst was delivery by mail and self-administration, as these had the lowest internal consistency reliability and also the lowest correlations with self-assessed dysfunction and illness.

Computer-based tests

The evidence suggests that computer-based tests can be effective. Velikova et al (2002) assessed computer-administered individual quality of life measurements in oncology clinics with immediate feedback of results to clinicians. The computer measurement was well accepted by patients, who felt that the questionnaires were a useful tool to tell the doctors about their problems, and clinicians felt that the data helped them identify issues for discussion as well as detect change over time.

Computer administration can also be reliable. Caro et al (2001) investigated whether electronic implementation of questionnaires lead to different results than paper versions. They found that collecting SF-36 and Asthma Quality of Life Questionnaire (AQLQ; Juniper et al 1992) data electronically reduced the number of spoiled responses without altering the results.

Computer-based presentation also allows adaptive testing (see Ch. 8 under 'Item Banking and Computer Adaptive Testing').

Outputs produced by the test

Consideration needs to be given to the outputs required from the test. It is generally desirable that instruments for measuring HQoL assess and report on a number of dimensions.

Providing dimension scores allows the instrument to play a diagnostic role, i.e. identify the areas of major concern. For example, in comparing the effectiveness of therapies there may be no clear advantage for one versus another when assessed globally. However, there could be differences in their profiles of effect, e.g. some dimensions improving, such as functional ability, and others becoming worse, e.g. more symptoms (Revicki 1989). It is useful to be able to examine dimension/subscale scores (see also Deyo & Patrick 1989, Donovan et al 1989, Goodinson & Singleton 1989, Bottomley 2002).

Meaningfulness or interpretability of the test result

Test results are not automatically meaningful. Further steps may be required to allow qualitative meaning to be assigned to the instrument's quantitative scores.

Issues in translating a quantitative score to a qualitative category that has clinical or commonly-understood meaning are discussed in Chapter 7 under 'Developing Interpretability', and Chapter 11 under 'Interpreting Quality of Life Scores for Individual Patients'.

Test development criteria

There is enormous variability in the way that tests are developed (see Ch. 9 under 'The Development of Some Generic Instruments'). The development method largely determines the ability of the test to carry out the required role. At the very least, the criteria should specify the *sources of information* necessary in gathering the content.

Content

Most tests are based on an identification and sampling of the domains relevant to the type of health state being assessed, and three sources of information should be consulted:

1. patients and their relatives
2. healthcare professionals experienced in the condition
3. the medical, behavioural, and social science literature.

If possible, an investigation should also be conducted to identify the nature of the content in terms of dimensions to be included. This can be conducted relatively easily via a search of the two literature databases *Index Medicus/Medline* and *PsychLit/PsychInfo* (there may also be relevant articles in health planning and health economics databases). Reports may be sought concerning:

- the illness/condition, and its effects as reported by patients, family members, and healthcare workers
- specific tests that claim to address the condition or related conditions, and generic tests that may play a role in assessing the condition.

In a thoughtful article discussing the 'ideal' HIV HQoL measure, Shumaker et al (1997) suggested that it was critical that the core dimensions of the test captured the issues that individuals targeted by the measure believed important (and to consider the full range of patient sub-populations).

Method of forming and scaling the test

A newcomer to the field would find it difficult to prepare criteria for this area. Test development encompasses many elements, such as the way scales or sub-scales are formed, e.g. sum scales based on Classical Test Theory versus Item Response Theory/Rasch models; the types of response scales that are used such as dichotomous, Likert, Guttman; the use of single items and tasks for gathering health state assessments; and methods of combining sub-scale scores.

Chapters 5, 6, and 7 should be read to develop an understanding of relevant issues.

Desired psychometric properties of the final test: validity, reliability, scaling

Criteria might also cover the psychometric properties of the test, although criteria here would require the most expertise to form.

In essence, a test that aims to measure HQoL is endeavouring to measure a construct. By construct is meant a hypothetical concept which can never be directly measured or absolutely confirmed, but only inferred from observations of behaviour. (Constructs also play a role in statistical techniques such as factor analysis, multiple regression, logistic regression, Item Response Theory, and structural equation models: for a discussion of such 'latent variables' see Bollen 2002.)

A test is a procedure for obtaining samples of the behaviour(s) and deriving numbers that estimate the value of the construct. This entails considering the legitimacy of the numbers, their reliability, validity, and scaling (see Crocker & Algina 1986, Anastasi 1990).

Problems facing the measurement of constructs are listed below, adapted from Crocker & Algina (1986). These issues are considered throughout this book. The problems faced are:

1. No single approach to the measurement of a construct (such as HQoL) is likely to be universally accepted. Measures of

psychological constructs are always indirect, hence theorists who talk about the construct may select very different behaviours to define the construct operationally. The stance adopted by the test developer needs to be made clear. The construct to be measured, and the purpose of the measure, need to be made clear (e.g. see earlier in this chapter, and Ch. 4).

2. Measurements are usually based on limited samples of behaviour – determining the number of items and the variety of content necessary to provide an adequate sample of the behavioural domain is a major problem in developing a sound measurement procedure (e.g. see Chs 4, 5, 6, 7, and 8).

3. The measurement obtained is always subject to error. It is very unlikely that re-testing of the same individuals would ever be identical, due to factors such as fatigue, boredom, guessing and carelessness (e.g. see Chs 6 and 8).

4. The measurement scales will often lack well-defined units – the properties of the measurement scale, the labelling of the units, and the interpretation of the values, need to be considered carefully (e.g. see Chs 5, 6 and 8).

5. The construct measured by the test must be both operationally defined (i.e. defined in terms of observable behaviour) and hence capable of being empirically demonstrated, and defined in terms of its relationship to other constructs or events in the real world (e.g. see Ch. 4 and Ch. 11 under 'Interpreting Quality of Life Scores for Individual Patients').

These issues are confronted by whoever develops a test and from whichever conceptual framework is used.

A SAMPLE SET OF CRITERIA

A sample set of criteria are presented in an appendix at the end of this chapter. These criteria are based on those used for the final development of the 'Work Ability Tables' (WATs), an expert-referenced test of work-related disability (O'Connor et al 1996; note that the WATs method of assessment is no longer used in the determination of Disability Support Pension eligibility).

APPENDIX

PRACTICAL NEEDS CRITERIA

1. The test should provide an overall score, plus sub-scores indicating work-related disability due to each of the domains (mobility, communication, etc.)
2. Able to be completed by a medical officer without special training following a routine medical examination
3. The form able to be completed within 5–10 minutes.

TEST DEVELOPMENT CRITERIA

1. The test should consist of a series of Guttman scales, with all Guttman response options scaled on the same metric of 'work-related disability' based on the ratings of an expert team of judges.
2. The team of judges used to rate items (in terms of work-related disability) need to possess the mix and range of skills necessary to estimate the effect of a disability on capacity to work.
3. The judges must have a clear and agreed conception regarding the judgements they are to make (i.e. need to clearly define 'ability to work').
4. The judges must be presented with items that reflect the nature of actual cases.
5. Within disability domains, the items must be clear, unambiguous and weighted so as to predict their contribution to disability arising within that domain. This means items within sub-scales must be independent.
6. All disability domains relevant to accurately assessing disability must be represented.
7. The disability domains that together form the overall scale must be weighted to allow valid representation of overall work-related disability.

DESIRED PSYCHOMETRIC PROPERTIES OF THE FINAL TEST

1. The test must be shown to exhibit inter-rater reliability, i.e. different medical officers should make the same assessment if

faced with a common patient (in terms of both descriptor selection and overall score).

2. The test score should correlate highly with unbiased clinical estimates of work-related disability (convergent validity).

3. The output of the test should correlate significantly with other measures of disability (convergent validity).

4. The test should be capable of clearly distinguishing between sub-populations of patients (discriminant validity).

5. The test should be capable of clearly distinguishing individuals within sub-populations of patients (sensitivity).

6. Ultimately, the test would ideally be examined for agreement with other indicators of validity. For example, of clients not granted disability status, did those with higher disability ratings show a greater tendency to not return to work/appear for reassessment/make an appeal, etc.?

SUMMARY

Specifying the purpose of a measure is necessary to ensure that the instrument is capable of performing the task demanded of it. A clear conceptualization of the construct (or concept) to be measured is also necessary.

Criteria should also be spelt out, as far as possible. The more criteria are specified at the beginning, the less effort will be wasted later.

KEY POINTS

First actions when selecting, assessing, developing or modifying a test, are to specify the following (as far as possible).

The purpose to which the test will be put, and the concept to be used (*essential*)

- What is the purpose of the test as defined by the test user?
- What is the attribute/ability to be measured?
- Where applicable, specify a criterion/proxy-criterion

Criteria the test needs to meet

- Practical needs criteria (*required*):
  - Size and time to complete
  - Interviewer versus self-administered tests

- Computer-based tests
- Outputs produced by the test
- Meaningfulness or interpretability of the test result
- Test Development criteria (*if possible*):
  - Content examined to form the test
  - Method of forming and scaling the test
- Desired psychometric properties of the final test (*if possible*):
  - Validity
  - Reliability
  - Scaling

4

Validity: the degree to which a scale measures what the user intends it to

AIMS OF CHAPTER

- To explain that:
  - validity refers to the use of a test, and is not a property of a test independently of its use – the test may be valid for one purpose, but not another
  - validity is a matter of degree, tests are not 'valid' or 'invalid'

- To describe the ways that validity can be assessed

- To describe the role of statistical techniques in assessing validity

- To emphasize that validity is the most important aspect of a test

With the rapidly increasing importance placed on health outcome measures, there have been a number of calls for greater attention to validity. Clancy & Lipscomb (2000) noted how rapid growth in the area 'make[s] us acutely aware of the need for clarity regarding what is really meant by validity', while Patrick & Chiang (2000a) referred to the challenge of ensuring that 'the validity of measures used in different applications and populations is well documented'. This chapter addresses these issues.

WHAT IS VALIDITY?

Paradoxically, while validity is the most fundamental issue in test application, it can be the least understood. The following endeavours to clear up some common misconceptions.

Tests are not valid, *uses* are (but only to a greater or lesser degree ...)

Validity refers to the degree to which a scale measures what the user intends it to measure.

Despite many books and articles over many years addressing what constitutes validity, the myth persists that a test is valid or invalid. This is emphatically not the case. There are no valid instruments per se. Validity applies to the *application* of an instrument, not to the instrument itself.

Moreover, validity is a matter of degree. The population to which the test will be applied is never identical to the population upon which it was developed, and the test will to some extent be less than perfect in carrying out its intended role. This is the case irrespective of the method used to develop the test.

Even those who advocate Rasch analysis on the grounds that it produces highly portable tests recognize that the tests are imperfect. 'Since the Rasch model is the expression of an unreachable (but essential and useful) ideal, no data ever fit it perfectly . . . (the process of refining the test) must stop when the measures are good enough for the purposes they are intended' (Linacre 1999).

To plan a validation study, the desired inference must be clearly identified and then evidence gathered. Validation is the process by which a test developer or test user collects evidence to support the type of inferences that are to be drawn from test scores (Crocker & Algina 1986 citing Cronbach 1971).

Validity is 'the degree to which evidence and theory support the interpretations of test scores entailed by proposed uses of tests' and 'It is the interpretations of test scores required by proposed uses that are evaluated, not the test itself. When test scores are used or interpreted in more than one way, each intended interpretation must be validated' (AERA et al 1999, p. 9).

All validity is construct validity

Construct validity refers to the 'whole' of validity theory, it includes content- and criterion-related validity. This view was articulated by Anastasi (1986, 1990), who argued that content-, criterion- and construct-related validation no longer corresponded to meaningfully distinct categories but were products of the developmental history of validation testing.

In Anastasi's view, test scores are *always* based on constructs. Even in a simple test, the factor being measured does not exactly correspond to a single empirical measure (e.g. in a test to measure an individual's walking speed, there would be a need to take representative measurements to obtain a distribution of speeds depending on context, purpose, the individual's condition at the time, etc.). See Anastasi (1990) and Anastasi & Urbina (1997).

Recognizing this, the 1999 Standards for Educational and Psychological Testing set aside the traditional division of validity into content, criterion and construct, and categorized validity evidence as follows:

A. Evidence based on test content (evaluation of suitability of content, i.e. content validity).
B. Evidence based on response processes (e.g. ways in which individuals respond when completing the test).
C. Evidence based on internal structure (inter-item relationships, factor analysis studies, and studies of differential item functioning).
D. Evidence based on relations to other variables (includes criterion-related validity).
E. Evidence based on the consequences of testing (e.g. descriptive studies of the extent to which anticipated benefits of testing are realized).

(1999 Standards for Educational and Psychological Testing; see Goodwin 2002)

Validity has become a unitary concept, it is the degree to which all of the accumulated evidence supports the intended interpretation of test scores for the intended purpose (AERA et al 1999, p. 11).

The terms content- and criterion-related validity will still be used in this book in referring to general areas to be considered (not discrete attributes of a test).

Validation is a continuing, critical and dynamic process

A stress on the need to actively critique tests is vital. This approach automatically proceeds once one accepts that validity refers to uses, not tests, and that validity is a matter of degree.

Validation should be a process of constructing and evaluating arguments for and against proposed test interpretations and uses . . . Instead of being advocates for the work we do, we are asked to embrace the scientific ideal of striving to understand and disclose the weaknesses as well as the strengths of our tests and testing practices. (Haertel in his presidential address at the annual meeting of the National Council on Measurement in Education, quoted by Goodwin 2002, p. 105.)

Validation as a continuing, critical, dynamic process is not always greatly in evidence. Potential users need to investigate tests thoroughly (see Ch. 10). In this respect, it is important that the characteristics of population samples used in validity-relevant research are always completely described, both in terms of variability, because this has such a large effect on correlational studies, and in terms of sub-groups that may or may not be present (i.e. limits on generalizability; see Mason et al 2003).

The following sections discuss a range of areas to consider when assessing or developing validity. The system roughly but not entirely follows the framework adopted by the 1999 Standards for Educational and Psychological Testing.

VALIDITY EVIDENCE BASED ON THE PROCESS OF CONSTRUCTION

If the process of test development is clear and rational, and the steps one would expect to be present *are* present, then the test is a priori likely to provide useful output. In other words, the primary determinant of an instrument's ability to measure is the process of construction ('Validity needs to be built into a test from the outset'; Anastasi 1990).

In a typical health-related quality of life (HQoL) test, the sampling of dimensions is central to validity: the domains that should be included depend upon the patients targeted. The number properties of the scale and sub-scales need also to be appropriate, and a suitable scoring algorithm developed. The process for constructing a classical test is discussed in Chapter 7.

VALIDITY EVIDENCE BASED ON TEST CONTENT
Ensuring tests include the right content

A major priority in constructing any test is to ensure that all the elements necessary to measure the construct have been included. Emphasis needs to be placed on ensuring that the instrument adequately assesses all the areas of the patient's life that are significantly affected by the condition or programme (i.e. 'content validity').

There is a need to identify the domains or categories of variables that are relevant before starting to assess the appropriateness of existing measures, and in general, assessment should examine factors that are likely to be affected by the intervention or have been troubling to patients in the past (Bergner 1989). Any failure to assess all relevant dimensions may lead to an inability to detect the impact of a treatment on quality of life (QoL) or to record no difference where one exists (Donovan et al 1989).

There should be a systematic examination of the test content to determine that it covers a representative sample of the behaviour domain to be measured. The items that form the test should convey the attribute, and also cover the full range of the attribute in a balanced way (with a multi-dimensional construct, there is likely to be a need to develop an appropriate weighting of these dimensions). The items need to adequately represent the performance domain or construct of specific interest.

Considerations include how separate elements are to be weighted and whether all elements necessary to represent the construct have been included. The domains should also be defined in advance rather than after the test has been prepared (Anastasi 1990).

WHICH DIMENSIONS SHOULD BE ASSESSED FOR A COMPREHENSIVE HEALTH-RELATED QUALITY OF LIFE TEST?

The dimensions that need to be assessed for a given test can only be determined by talking to the patients, their families and friends, healthcare workers, and by examining the literature.

Revicki et al (2000) observed that most claims for treatment-related HQoL benefits for new pharmaceutical and medical devices were restricted to demonstrated differences on one or several HQoL domains. Revicki et al pointed out that this would not indicate overall HQoL benefit unless there was also evidence that the domains were those that individuals with a specific disease valued as important to their HQoL.

The dimensions that are relevant also depend on the purpose of the test. In considering the effectiveness of care programmes for chronically ill, home-based patients, there is a strong case for assessing the HQoL of other family members, i.e. those who may have to provide the major care and who may themselves be aged or infirm.

The domains to include may vary with different stages of the same illness. Berzon et al (1997) reported nine dimensions relevant to assessing the effects of early human immunodeficiency virus (HIV) disease.

The process of identifying additional content for tests should be ongoing. Silberfeld et al (2002) interviewed dementia patients and their care givers to identify aspects of QoL perceived as relevant and important, and then compared respondent report with the content of three generic utility-based QoL instruments. They concluded that essential attributes of dementia QoL identified by the respondents were missing in each of the three instruments examined. Others have identified the need for additional domains to measure social outcomes in disability and rehabilitation research (Dijkers et al 2000), and a new cognitive domain for the EQ-5D questionnaire (classification system for the description of health states developed by the EuroQol Group [EuroQol Group 1990, Brooks 1996]) (Krabbe et al 1999).

Studies that have systematically examined the importance of different aspects of health-related QoL have produced interesting results. Hall et al (1989) explored the perceptions of elderly people to determine the relationship among various domains of health, in the sense of health being perceived as a multidimensional construct, and the degree to which patient perceptions of their own health corresponded to the perceptions of their physicians. The results suggested that 'social support of the non-family kind' was a variable of the order of importance of functional health in indicating subjective well-being. As restricted social activity can be both a consequence of illness conditions and possibly play a major role in determining subjective well-being, 'non-family social support' may be a desirable dimension in tests estimating the effects of health on QoL.

In summary, there is a need for the systematic exploration of the range of domains for a given condition, the relative importance of different domains, and the identification of any interactions between domains.

As indicated in Chapter 2, there may also be a place for identifying and including variables that predict conditions under which psychological adaptation will fail and lead to diminished well-being.

'Descriptive validity'

'Descriptive validity' refers to the ability of an instrument to comprehensively characterize a patient's health status (Bergner et al 1981). Bergner argued that items should be retained in the Sickness Impact Profile (SIP) even if they failed to account for additional variance, on the grounds that they contribute to the descriptive capacity of the SIP (see Ch. 9). This useful notion opposes the common wish to simplify measures.

VALIDITY EVIDENCE RELATED TO THE TEST TASKS

An important consideration is whether the test tasks produce elements that interfere with measurement of the test construct, by introducing complex performance elements.

Some tasks, such as are sometimes used in health utility measurement, seem overly complex. The assumptions underlying these methods were challenged by Kaplan et al (1993), who noted that human information processors do poorly at integrating complex probability information when making decisions that involve risk (as is required in many utility measurement tasks). Similarly Lenert & Kaplan (2000) argued that utility measures could introduce construct-irrelevant variance due to their elicitation methods.

These issues are discussed further in Chapter 11, 'Measuring Utilities'.

VALIDITY EVIDENCE BASED ON RELATIONS TO OTHER VARIABLES

Types of comparison

There are many types of validity assessment based on relationships between test scores and other variables. The 1999 Standards for Educational and Psychological Testing (see Goodwin 2002) listed these as:

1. Correlational studies of the type and extent of relationships between scores and external variables.
2. Correlational studies of the extent to which scores forecast or predict criterion performance or scores on measures obtained at a later date.
3. Convergent validity studies, investigating the relationships between scores and other tests intended to measure similar constructs.
4. Discriminant validity studies, investigating the relationships between scores and other measures of purportedly different constructs.
5. Experimental studies, intended to test hypotheses about effects of specific interventions on test scores.
6. Known-group comparison studies, intended to test hypotheses about expected differences in test scores across specific groups of examinees.
7. Studies of the effectiveness of selection, placement, and classification decisions.
8. Differential group prediction or relationship studies.
9. Studies of validity generalization.

The most common types of test score-other variable comparisons when assessing health outcome measures are as follows.

Known-group comparison studies.   In this commonly used form, individuals or populations hypothesized to differ on the test construct are assessed using the test. If the expected differences are found, the test is supported.

Correlations between the test and other tests.   This more dubious category requires that correlations be moderately high but not too high, for otherwise, the new test represents needless duplication (unless the other test is less convenient to use).

Correlation between the test and external variables.   Assessment of the test's capacity to correlate with external variables such as institutionalization, readmission, use of services, etc.

Correlation between test score and a criterion.   See Criterion-related Validity below.

Longitudinal studies assessing the effects of disease course or treatment.   See Responsiveness below.

Responsiveness

A HQoL measure needs to be able to discriminate between levels of a disease condition due to disease course or treatment, which is commonly termed 'responsiveness' meaning sensitivity to change. Some have suggested that this represents a separate issue to reliability and validity (e.g. Deyo & Patrick 1989), but the view adopted here is that 'sensitivity/responsiveness' is part of validity (as has been argued by others, e.g. Terwee et al 2003).

If an instrument is markedly lacking in 'responsiveness', it may exhibit floor and/or ceiling effects, i.e. failure to detect a worsening state in patients who already have a poor QoL (floor effect), or improvement for patients whose QoL is relatively good (ceiling effect). See Higginson & Carr (2001).

For a review of frequently used responsiveness statistics, see Husted et al (2000).

Birbeck et al (2000) noted that a barrier to the use of HQoL measures in clinical trials is the dearth of information regarding the responsiveness of existing measures to changes in clinical status, and Liang (2000) pointed out that there are few studies that evaluate the extent to which health status or HQoL measures capture clinically important changes. See also Dempster et al (2002).

The issue of responsiveness overlaps with that of clinical meaningfulness. See Chapter 11 under 'Interpreting Quality of Life Scores for Individual Patients'.

Criterion-related validity

Criterion-related validation indicates the effectiveness of a test in predicting an individual's specified performance or report. It entails performance on the test being checked against a 'criterion', that is *a direct and independent measure of the variable the test is designed to predict* (Anastasi 1990, Anastasi & Urbina 1997). Validity can be estimated based on the correlation coefficient between predictor and criterion scores.

With criterion-related validity, the behaviour of interest can be directly measured. The scale is necessary because either/or:

- a test is quicker, simpler, or less expensive (concurrent validity)
- the behaviour could only be determined in the future (predictive validity)
- a multi-item test is desired for greater reliability
- a test is needed that can both predict the criterion and estimate the factors responsible for any change in the criterion (i.e. provide sub-scale values).

Criteria may come from personal judgement by those considered expert in the area. Such experts may provide categorical judgements (e.g. a diagnosis), or quantitative estimates via ratings. In this respect, Anastasi noted that ratings have been employed in the validation of almost every type of test, and when obtained under carefully controlled conditions with adequately trained raters, represent a valuable source of criterion data (Anastasi 1990, pp. 645–647).

Validity coefficient

Calculating the correlation between a test score and a criterion (a direct and independent measure of the variable the test is designed to predict) forms a *validity coefficient*. The Pearson Product-Moment Correlation can be used for this.

The validity coefficient may also be interpreted as the *standard error of estimate*, analogous to the error of measurement in connection with reliability. Even with a validity of 0.80, the error of predicted scores may be considerable, but a test may improve predictive efficiency if it shows any significant correlation with the criterion, however low. Anastasi (1990) suggests that even validities as low as 0.20 or 0.30 may justify use of the test, depending on the relative benefit from having the test.

Criterion measures in health

It is sometimes argued that criterion validity is not possible for a *broad* health status measure because no criterion exists that accurately measures the phenomena of interest (Kaplan et al 1976). Similarly, Aaronson et al (2002) maintained that in self-reported health status assessment, criterion-related validity is rarely tested 'because of the absence of widely accepted criterion measures'.

In the view of the author, this position is not sustainable. Tests that aim to estimate, e.g. the QoL of patients, do have a criterion source – the reports of the patients themselves. For each possible application of the test, there is likely to be a group of patients from whom a criterion measure can be gathered.

In fact, criterions are widely used in the development of HQoL tests. A faultless criterion does not exist (there may never be a single empirical measure that exactly corresponds to the construct), but there is frequently a measure close to being a criterion (or 'proxy-criterion').

See Chapter 5 under 'Patient Global Self Ratings' and 'Global Ratings as Criterion Measures in Test Development' for further discussion of criterions.

The Multitrait-Multimethod Matrix method

The Multitrait-Multimethod Matrix framework for convergent and discriminant validation was put forward by Campbell & Fiske (1959), who proposed that a test should correlate highly with variables it would be theoretically expected to, and not correlate highly with variables with which it would be expected to differ. The systematic method entails the assessment of two or more constructs by two or more methods. For details see Campbell & Fiske (1959) and Anastasi & Urbina (1997).

VALIDITY EVIDENCE BASED ON INTERNAL STRUCTURE

Evidence of internal consistency and/or item order

Test models generally require that items represent a (specified) unidimensional construct (at least within sub-scales). Evidence of this is seen to support the validity of the test.

High inter-item and item-total correlations among test items can be interpreted as evidence that the items measure a single construct (based on Classical Test Theory; see Ch. 6 under 'The Sum Scale Approach of Classical Test Theory').

Evidence that items are ordered as expected, given the nature of the construct, may also be used to support the test (based on Item Response Theory [IRT]; see Ch. 8 under 'The Rasch Model').

Such 'internal to the test' characteristics do not, however, confirm that the test is measuring what is desired; data external to the test are necessary. Salzberger (2000) recently stressed the limitations of pursuing validity based on the internal structure of the construct, but not related to criteria outside the construct, in the context of developing trans-cultural tests. Others generally urge caution (e.g. Anastasi & Urbina 1997).

> **The contribution of validity evidence based on internal structure is limited. Data external to the test itself are more important.**

The role of factor analysis

Factor analysis can be used as a more sophisticated means of examining item inter-correlations. Factor analysis involves obtaining a range of 'n' measures (items) on the same testees, then computing an $n \times n$ correlation matrix. Underlying variables or 'factors' are then sought to account for the patterns of correlation between the measures. It can be determined whether the items cluster together as predicted by the theoretical structure of the construct (see Anastasi & Urbina 1997).

A number of researchers have stressed caution in the use of exploratory factor analysis. Kaplan et al (1976) opposed factor analysis as a tool in the development of health status indexes, arguing that once factor analysis derived underlying factors based on groups of items, items checked rarely or poorly correlated with others would be considered unimportant and tend to be excluded. Kaplan et al argued that such items might correspond to rare conditions, which while not loading significantly on any of the larger factors and not representing a substantial unique factor were, nonetheless, extremely important for the proper assessment of those rare cases (cf. Bergner's notion of 'descriptive validity'). There are further criticisms, e.g. that factors are unstable and highly sample dependent, and can be generated as artifacts when there is a large range of item difficulties. In this respect, it is important to stress again that items should not be rejected, or accepted, solely on statistical grounds. Both logic and empiricism must play a role when developing measures of constructs (Anastasi 1986).

Nonetheless, factor analysis is extensively used. For example, Devins et al (2001) examined the Illness Intrusiveness Ratings Scale (IIRS) to determine whether a common underlying factor structure existed across different patient populations, to justify comparing IIRS scores within or between groups. See also Hall et al (1989) and Coyne et al (2002).

A related and more respected procedure is *confirmatory factor analysis* or, more generally, structural equation modelling (see MacCallum & Austin 2000), which tests whether latent variables are linearly inter-related in a way that would be expected, given hypothesized relationships. The implications of the proposed inter-relationships are determined for the variances and covariances of the variables, and the actual fit of the data to the model is then examined. For examples of the application of structural equation modelling, see Crowley & Fan (1997), Keller et al (1998a), Power et al (1999), Carlsson & Hamrin (2002) and Bjorner et al (2003).

See Nunnally & Bernstein (1994) for further details of exploratory and confirmatory factor analysis.

CORRELATION AND REGRESSION
Interpreting correlation coefficients

As with correlation coefficients generally, sample heterogeneity is a major influence. Restriction of variance in the scores of X or Y variables can reduce the maximum correlation value that can be obtained. The wider the range of scores, the higher will be the correlation.

Crocker & Algina (1986) suggest that whenever a low correlation coefficient is obtained, the researcher should determine whether a restriction in variance has occurred because of sample selection or some aspect of the measurement process. Examining the bivariate distribution via a scatter plot is recommended. Examining the scatterplot will also reveal if the relationship is linear and uniform, as the Pearson Product-Moment Correlation assumes equal variability throughout the range (i.e. homeoscedasticity; see Shavelson 1988).

In interpreting correlation coefficients, the magnitude of the coefficient needs to be checked against the two criteria of whether it is significantly different from 0.00, and what percentage of variance in one variable is shared with variance in the other (see Hays 1981, Shavelson 1988). Remember also that high correlations between variables does not mean that they are causally related, as some further intervening variable may affect both variables.

It is particularly important to be aware that high correlations can conceal important differences. Bergner et al (1976b) demonstrated that an overall moderate or high correlation may mask shortcomings in sensitivity for particular sub-groups. They found the correlation for a total subject sample between self-assessment of dysfunction and SIP score to be 0.52. This was more than each of several sub-groups alone, with the correlations for one sub-group (speech pathology patients) being −0.01.

The role of multiple regression in health-related quality of life measurement

Multiple regression (MR) has a long history of use in the development and validation of health status measures for the prediction of health status (e.g. Lipscomb 1989, Hall et al 1989). Logistic regression in which the dependent variable has only two possible outcomes is also popular.

Multiple regression can be of particular use where there is multidimensionality of the construct (Anastasi 1990, Anastasi & Urbina 1997). This can lead to the development of a number of unidimensional sub-tests, rather than a single test consisting of many different sorts of items. This allows a clear assessment of relevant dimensions, and maintains reliability within sub-tests.

It is often preferable to use a combination of several relatively homogeneous tests, each covering a different aspect of the criterion, rather than a single test consisting of a hodgepodge of many different kinds of items (Anastasi & Urbina 1997).

The combination of HQoL sub-tests to allow a single global estimate can then be achieved by multiple regression against a criterion. Alternatively, it is possible to gather a global estimate using one or more items dedicated to this purpose, and it has been argued elsewhere that this is still a good idea (a direct measure of self-assessed global HQoL may, for example, allow adaptation to be estimated). However, multiple regression against a criterion (such as self-assessed global HQoL) allows the relative importance of the unidimensional domains to be determined.

For example, Bernheim (1999) advocated the use of such a method with the Anamnestic Comparative Self Assessment tool (ACSA), where subjects first define their individual scales of QoL with poles of the best and the worst times in their lives and then locate their current health status on these scales. The weights of the dimensions in the multi-item questionnaire were to be determined through regression against global self-assessment (both multiple items and a global question were required).

Note that sub-tests that correlate highly with each other represent statistical duplication. One of two highly correlated tests would serve about as effectively as the pair in terms of predicting a criterion. However, both may need to be retained in the test to maintain its appearance as balanced and appropriate ('face validity') and to provide a clear clinical characterization of the patient.

Caution is needed when using multiple regression. Many independent variables (e.g. sub-scales) can be easily generated and selection of independent variables based on grounds other than simple empiricism is essential. One approach is to identify items based on the literature and discussions with patients and care givers, and to cluster them into a small number of dimensions as appropriate. Step-wise regression might then be used to identify the sub-scale dimensions that will form a possible model, followed by best sub-sets regression to check that an alternative model with the same number of independent variables is not more suitable (see Thompson 1995, for cautions against relying solely on step-wise regression).

A related caution is that the multiple correlation between the criterion and sub-tests indicates the highest predictive value that can be obtained, when each sub-scale is given optimum weight for predicting the criterion in question. These weights are optimal only for the particular sample in which they were derived. It is important that the test algorithm is cross-validated by correlating the predicted criterion scores with the actual criterion scores in a new sample. Formulas are available to estimate shrinkage in a multiple correlation; the larger the original sample the smaller the shrinkage, but empirical verification is considered preferable.

Experimentalists have in the past criticized multiple regression as an inferior statistic, particularly in comparison to analysis of variance (ANOVA). However, Cohen (1968) argued that MR is a far more powerful and flexible analytical system. Dummy variables allow the coding of nominal scale data, subtle variables can be captured via contrast coding, and curvilinear relationships can be examined by means of a polynomial form in power terms so that non-linear regression can be represented within the linear multiple regression framework. The preference for ANOVA was proposed as in part reflecting the original non-availability of MR, because it requires the computation and inversion of a matrix of correlations (or sums of squares and products) among the independent variables which require major computation for even a few independent variables. With modern electronic data processing there is no longer a barrier.

Anderson (1976) has pointed out that regression-correlation methodology can be useful in applied prediction, but can be misleading when it comes to testing theoretical models. Indeed, the great usefulness of regression-correlation analysis in applied prediction stems largely from its insensitivity to real deviations from linear summation models.

For further discussion of the use of multiple regression in aggregating sub-tests, see Anastasi & Urbina (1997, pp. 156–158). Criterions in HQoL assessment are discussed further in Chapter 5 under 'Patient Global Self-ratings' and 'Global Ratings as Criterion Measures in Test Development'. See also Chapter 7 under 'Developing a Method for Combining Sub-test Scores'.

SUMMARY

The nature of validity

- Tests are not valid, **uses** are. Validity applies to the application of an instrument, not to the instrument itself, and validity is a matter of degree (tests/applications are not 'valid' or 'invalid').
- All validity is construct validity. Validity is the degree to which all of the accumulated evidence supports the intended interpretation of test scores for the intended purpose.
- Validation is a continuing, critical, dynamic process. Potential users need to investigate tests thoroughly for themselves.

Validity evidence based on the process of construction

- If the process of test development is clear and rational, and the steps one would expect *are* present, then the test is a priori likely to provide useful output.

Validity evidence based on test content ('content validity')

- Items should convey the attribute and cover the full range of the attribute in a balanced way (with a multidimensional test; there also needs to be appropriate weighting of the dimensions). The dimensions to be included depend on the purpose of the test and talks with patients, their families and friends, healthcare workers, and the literature.
- The ability of an instrument to comprehensively characterize a patient's health status is a valuable and useful notion that opposes the common wish to simplify measures ('descriptive validity').

Validity evidence related to the test tasks

- An important consideration is whether the test tasks produce elements that interfere with measurement of the test construct, by introducing complex performance elements (particularly a concern with some utility tasks).

Validity evidence based on relations to other variables

- Correlations between the test and other tests, known groups studies, correlation with external variables.
- Responsiveness – sensitivity to change due to disease course or treatment.
- Criterion-related validity – performance on the test being checked against a criterion, i.e. a direct and independent measure of that which the test is designed to predict.

Validity evidence based on internal structure

- Evidence of high inter-item and item-total correlations (Classical Test Theory tests), and/or items spread along a continuum in an ordered manner (for IRT/Rasch models).
- Evidence from factor analysis of whether items cluster together as predicted by the theoretical structure of the construct.

Correlation and regression

When assessing validity by correlating a test score and another measure:
- The wider the range of scores, the higher will be the correlation. If a low correlation coefficient is obtained, the

researcher should determine whether a restriction in variance has occurred, e.g. through sample selection.

- The magnitude of the coefficient needs to be checked against the two criteria of whether it is significantly different from 0.00, and what percentage of variance in one variable is shared with variance in the other.
- Be aware that high correlations for populations can conceal low correlations for population sub-groups.

Multiple regression (and logistic regression)

- Can be used to combine several homogeneous sub-tests to form an index of HQoL as the superordinate construct and to determine the relative importance of the sub-tests/domains.

KEY POINTS

- Validity is the most fundamental issue in test application. *Tests are not valid, applications are, and only to a degree*. Potential users need to investigate tests thoroughly for themselves.
- The primary determinant of an instrument's ability to measure accurately what it is intended to measure is the process of construction. Validity needs to be built into a test from the outset. After defining what is to be estimated and the purpose of the instrument is specified, the sampling of the proper dimensions is central to validity.
- For example, when measuring HQoL, the domains that are particularly relevant depend upon the patient's illness. The number properties of the scale and sub-scales need also to be tested, which generally means items in different domains need to be scaled using the same measure. Finally, sub-scales/domains need to be weighted and/or a scoring algorithm developed to ensure the output of the test properly reflects the impact of scores in multiple domains.
- Finally, and most importantly, there should be correlation of scores with external real-life criteria. This needs to be combined with *very* close examination of the results of such correlation analyses, to ensure that an overall high correlations is not masking a major failure of the instrument for important sub-groups. This is particularly relevant when validating generic health status measures, given the range of patient types that they are required to handle.

5

Single-item measures for scaling health states

AIMS OF CHAPTER

- To introduce the background of attempts to quantify health states, and the development of the rating tasks commonly used to make global assessments

- To indicate the manner and extent to which task factors can influence estimates

- To reveal that single item tasks can provide estimates comparable to the output of multi-item scales

- To indicate the important role patient global self-ratings play in health outcome measurement

- To indicate the value of single item global measures as criterions

THE BACKGROUND OF SCALING IN PSYCHOPHYSICS

Scaling refers to 'the theory and practice of associating numbers with psychological objects' (Eyfuth 1972).

The origins of scaling lie in early psychophysics, the 'manner in which living organisms respond to the energetic configurations of the environment' (Stevens 1972). Psychophysics was largely concerned with efforts to determine the functional relationship between a physical stimulus and perceptual experience, e.g. how loud a sound was reported to be, versus a physical measure of the sound intensity. The methods that arose from these investigations have since been applied to the scaling of attitudes or abilities, including perceptions and experiences of health states.

Category rating, magnitude rating and equivalence rating

The early psychophysicists were concerned to study the relationship between measurement of the same property obtained in two different ways, e.g. the relationship between weight, length and temperature defined by the response of human subjects as instruments, and weight, length and temperature defined by other measuring instruments such as scales, rules, and thermometers. A psychophysical law is a statement of the relationship between measurements obtained by these two methods. The experimental methods and statistical processes developed by the early psychophysicists were later applied to measure human ability, personality, attitudes, etc.

In what became a classical work, Stevens (e.g. see Stevens & Galanter 1957) divided stimuli into those forming quantitative ('prothetic'), and qualitative ('metathetic') continua. Prothetic continua were seen to be concerned with 'how much', i.e. quantitative aspects. An example is loudness, where different levels were formed by adding more of the same. Metathetic continua were concerned with 'what kind', or 'where', i.e. qualitative aspects. An example is pitch, where differences are due to the substitution of new frequencies for old.

Stevens described the main differences between prothetic and metathetic continua as being exhibited in the formal relations that could be observed among three primary kinds of scaling measures, i.e. partition, magnitude, and confusion measures.

- *Category rating.* With partition scales (category scales) the observer assigns one of a finite set of numbers to each stimulus, e.g. the numbers one to five, or adjectives such as small, medium, large. This is seen to represent judgements of subjective differences, or distances.
- *Magnitude rating.* In magnitude scales, the observer is asked to directly assign numbers to stimuli in proportion to their apparent magnitude, or of ratios among apparent magnitudes (the function relating stimulus magnitude to subjective magnitude is generally determined to be a power one).
- *Equivalence tasks.* These tasks tend to be concerned with issues of determining thresholds of no difference/difference, with scales such as JND (just noticeable difference), discrimination, paired comparisons and successive intervals.

Stevens found that on quantitative continua, *partition* scaling methods are usually curved relative to the *magnitude* scale. With qualitative continua, scaling methods are linearly related (the loss of linearity between methods was seen by Stevens as being a product of forcing the observer to partition the continuum, and prevent the making of a proportional number assignment that would preserve ratios: this restriction causes the dramatic curvature in the scale). With quantitative continua, *confusion scales* were reported to be logarithmically related to magnitude scales, while being linear on metathetic continua.

No scaling is direct: there are effects of instructions, stimuli and response

Initially, magnitude estimation was the method of choice for scaling psychophysical functions, but there has since been a retreat from that view. In a major review of psychophysical scaling, Gescheider (1988) concluded that sensation magnitude cannot be measured directly by any method, including methods that require subjects to assign numbers to stimuli that presumably represent sensation magnitude (e.g. magnitude estimation or category scaling).

Responses in the scaling task came to be seen as a joint function of cognitive and sensory factors, first a sensory stage and then a cognitive stage. While average magnitude estimations were approximately a power function of stimulus intensity, subjects responses were influenced by many stimulus variables, e.g. the range of stimuli presented in the experiment. Results suggested that subjects rehearsed the psychological continuum in which the stimulus was presented, with their response determined by the perceived location of the stimulus on the continuum relative to various possible anchors.

It was apparent that responses in psychophysical experiments could be biased in many ways. Which effects appeared (some biases were contradictory) seemed dependent upon subtle conditions of *instructions*, *stimuli*, and *response*, including:

- Instruction or 'framing' effects: e.g. where numerical examples were given in magnitude estimation tasks, the function was found to vary depending on the size of the numerical ratio given as an example.
- Stimulus frequency bias: stimuli presented that are a little larger or smaller than a frequently presented stimulus are judged to be excessively different.
- Sequential bias effects: a bias to report values similar to the last reported (successive measures are correlated) – this reduced the response range, through assimilation of the responses toward the centre.
- Contraction bias: subjects' responses are closer to the centre of the response range than they should be.
- The tendency to use categories equally often in category rating.
- Stimulus equalization bias: the tendency to use the full range of responses whatever the size of the range of the stimuli.

(See Gescheider 1988.)

Category rating and magnitude estimation may measure different things

With the growth of cognitive psychology there came an emphasis upon cognitive processes as determinants of perception and response. As *both* category scaling and magnitude estimation appeared to pass a variety of interval-scaling tests, it was suggested each procedure produced valid measurements of different psychological processes. Perhaps sensory magnitudes and sensory dissimilarities of stimuli were equally meaningful but different dimensions of experience (Gescheider 1988).

ISSUES WHEN SCALING HEALTH STATES

Psychophysics was the primary model for initial health state scaling studies. Of course for health states, one cannot *present* the experience of ill health to subjects (unlike when scaling, say, illumination where one can present a range of lights and determine a subject's ability to discriminate among them and estimate differences). Either one uses a range of patients who have experienced different states and use a common measuring tool, or a single group of subjects and ask them to rate a description.

Rating scales can be made easy to understand

The developers of the Quality of Well-Being index or QWB (e.g. see Kaplan et al 1989) invested significant effort in attempting to determine the characteristics of different scaling procedures, particularly the merits of a category rating scale, now more commonly referred to as (simply) a 'rating scale'.

A range of studies comparing variants of the psychophysical category rating, magnitude estimation and equivalence tasks (Patrick et al 1973, Kaplan et al 1979, Kind & Rosser 1988) gave conflicting results, although a logarithmic relationship was reported between values obtained via category rating versus magnitude estimation (Kaplan et al 1979; similarly Kind & Rosser 1988). An influential variable seemed to be the presence of defined end-points on a response scale, possibly the most distinguishing feature of a 'category rating' as opposed to a 'magnitude estimation' task (i.e. clearly defining the boundaries of the scale may be more important than whether the subject estimates stimulus values in terms of ratios or differences).

One useful feature of the category rating task (now 'rating scale') is that it allows the use of simple visual aids to help understand the task, i.e. when it is presented as a visual analogue scale (VAS). Brooks (1991) observed that perhaps the most attractive feature of category rating was 'the visual nature of the approach, which can help raters conceptualise what is required of them in evaluating health states' (Brooks 1991, p. 19).

Of course a category rating/rating scale does not require a visual scale, i.e. a task can seek interval-type judgments on a clearly bounded scale without reference to a visual aid. As pointed out earlier, terms can be confusing and misleading. It is essential to describe the task in all its features.

Further evidence favouring well-defined scale end-points

There are good grounds for supporting a scale with well-defined end-points. The evidence comes from investigations by Kaplan & Ernst (1983) of the reported tendency for distribution effects in category rating tasks, i.e. that subjects tend to spread their responses across all the allowable categories (Stevens & Galanter 1957, Parducci 1968). Kaplan & Ernst conducted experiments to investigate whether or not and under what conditions distribution effects occurred.

In their first experiment, Kaplan & Ernst used a 10-point rating scale, and instructions that included descriptions of a completely well person and a person in a coma so as to define clearly the end-points of the scale. Different groups of subjects were presented with four different groups of health state scenarios: all high scale items, all low, all medium, and mixed. Analysis of the ratings of health state descriptions by subjects who saw only high scale values produced some evidence of distribution effects. There was a slight trend for these subjects to spread their ratings of high items across the response range (from 0 'as bad as dying' to 10 'completely well') relative to the assignment of the same sub-set of high scale items by different subjects who were presented with the high sub-set in the context of a broader overall range of items. This trend was not supported in a second experiment.

However, a further experiment suggested that such effects could occur under conditions where subjects did not have or were not given clear information regarding the types of items that should define the end-points of the scale. In this experiment, subjects were to assess acts of immorality, and those subjects given instructions that clearly defined the end-points *did* produce responses distributed differently to those given minimal instructions.

Kaplan & Ernst concluded from this that health state assessments using a scale with well-defined poles were resistant to context effects. To minimize context effects of the distribution type it was suggested that:

- the continuum along which states are to be rated should be well-defined
- the end-points should be clearly defined
- the stimuli should not be available for inspection prior to their rating.

To this might be added the provision of enough scale points to allow maximum discrimination between judgements.

The provision of uncertain end-points to a scale may lead category rating to produce ordinal scales. For example, Read et al (1984) appeared to require subjects to define the extremes of the scale themselves, picking the worst and best outcomes (where the best was not a state of perfect health), and then filling in the medium values. This explicit requirement to use all the values of the scale would seem to counteract its 'absolute' nature, i.e. it encourages subjects to make relative selections of scale points.

A related issue concerns the zero point. There are states judged worse than death (see Ch. 11 under 'Measuring Utilities'), which poses problems in clearly defining the poles (see Sutherland et al 1983). This point was indirectly addressed by Haig et al (1986) who inverted the traditional poles of the illness–health continuum in a magnitude rating task, such that the *absence* of dysfunction or discomfort became zero, with the other end of the scale undefined. This is not a satisfactory option for category rating, seeming to solve one problem (death was no longer zero), but creating another (perfect health = ?).

Overall, context effects can be minimized by the use of rating scales where there has been careful definition of both the end-points and the continuum. Rating scales seem best anchored with clearly defined and operationalized end-points, and death not included. Visual rating scales are well supported.

Operationalize terms

In scaling generally, where terms such as 'frequently', 'seldom', or 'hardly ever', are used, anchoring by specifying the meaning of each response option will tend to reduce error variance. Thus 'hardly ever' can become 'once a month or less', seldom becomes 'at least once a month' and 'frequently' becomes 'weekly'. The actual anchors need to be determined through pre-testing (Nunnally & Bernstein 1994).

Avoid overly complex tasks

If one wishes to minimize the influence of complex cognitive variables, e.g. task complexity, and focus on the aspect of interest, e.g. desirability or otherwise of a health state, then it is sensible to use a task that is as simple as possible. The rating task seems to satisfy this condition.

For example, Patrick et al (1973) found that both category and magnitude estimation procedures were easy to use, as opposed to the method of equivalent stimuli which was complex, and reported to be 'unrealistic, emotive, confusing, and offensive to some judges' (consistent with this, the equivalence or tradeoff method also tended to give the largest standard deviations). Later evidence suggested that the magnitude estimation task was not clearly understood by subjects (Kaplan & Ernst 1983). Most recently, Saigal et al (2001) found that 16% of patients were unable to comprehend the time tradeoff task well enough to have utilities elicited.

One study did report category scaling as harder to use than the seemingly much more complex standard gamble or time tradeoff; however, in this study, a subject was asked to mark on a VAS the relative desirability of comprehensive health state descriptions using three marks – one for 3 months left to live, one for 8 years, and one for normal life expectancy (Torrance 1976). This task required the subject to estimate and combine QoL per state and length of time simultaneously (Kaplan et al 1976 suggested the result was due to item complexity and because the category rating task was presented first). This example illustrates the importance of looking at the whole task, not just some abstracted element of it.

Complex tasks should be avoided so as to focus on the primary aspect of interest, the perception or experience of a health state. For further discussion see 'Cautions When Using Single Item Tests' later in this chapter.

Be aware of framing effects

There is ample evidence that the set-up of a test or items may encourage testees to respond in a particular way, i.e. 'framing effects'. Framing effects are indicated when subjects make different decisions when presented with essentially the same information but different reference points (Tversky & Kahneman 1981, McNeil et al 1982).

Cohen et al (1996) examined sensitivity to wording in assessing patient satisfaction, and found responses were more likely to indicate greater satisfaction when patients were asked to agree/disagree with a negative description of their hospital experience than with a positive description. Fahey et al (1995) described how different methods of presenting results to health authority purchasers from a clinical trial and systematic review lead to differences in willingness to purchase services.

Llewelyn-Thomas et al (1984) examined the effect on numerical values assigned to health states of presenting a written description in formalized point form as used in the development of the Index of Well-being (Patrick et al 1973), versus scenarios similar in style to that used by Torrance (written in detail in the first person singular in common language), and found the point form scenarios produced higher values. See also Mellers et al (1998).

The nature of the item frame is very important: testees respond in different ways when presented with essentially the same information but different references and formats.

PATIENT GLOBAL SELF-RATINGS

Simple, single-item global questions asked of patients can be valid and sensitive, and play a key role as outcome measures in their own right, as well as in test development.

This is despite that fact that the estimates of HQoL are most commonly obtained using multi-item tests, either of the sum-scale type (Ch. 6) or using latent trait theory (Ch. 8).

Uses of patient global self-ratings

Uses of patient global self-ratings are as follows.

To estimate overall health-related quality of life

Global measures are often gathered from patients to make sense of complex treatment and illness effects. Feinstein (1999) observed that 'clinimetric global ratings' are frequently used as a gold standard when the US Food and Drug Administration evaluates diverse outcomes after treatment, and when psychometricians and statisticians seek a criterion with which to appraise criterion validity for a summated multicomponent score.

For example, Birbeck et al (2000) used a global patient report when endeavouring to assess the responsiveness (defined as ability to detect change over time) of various tests for epilepsy. This arose through concern that measures such as seizure counts did not capture a broad range of outcomes that may be relevant in evaluating the clinical impact of the many medical and surgical interventions now used. Birbeck et al asked subjects about their overall QoL at baseline and follow-up. They provided a graded set of response options and the question: 'We would like you to think about the present time. Please rate your overall condition as it is now, at this time. This rating should encompass factors such as social activities, performance at work or school, seizures, alertness, and functional capacity, that is, your overall quality of life'.

To allow individualized direct report

Feinstein has argued strongly that simple direct clinical questions (e.g. How are you? Are you better? How is the quality of your life?) may sometimes be more valuable and informative than the 'summated score of a horde of validated items' (Feinstein 1999).

Wright (2000) observed that clinicians do not usually rely on health status questionnaires to judge the success of therapy, but ask patients directly if they are better. Wright argues that patients come to their doctors with unique, different, and individual concerns, and their report should be able to convey this (Wright argued for a battery of individualized items, but patient-reported global estimates of HQoL also allows a free, direct report).

Similarly, Pugh-Clarke et al (2002) argued that the fixed nature of HQoL instruments is problematic, in that what is measured is predetermined and hence may not represent the free choice of the individual whose QoL is assessed – questionnaire-based instruments may not reflect individual priorities (see also Ruta et al 1999, and the patient generated index of quality of life or PGI).

With this same orientation, Bernheim (1999) argued for the value of the 'How have you been?' question because it entailed global self-assessment. Bernheim maintains that while multiple dimensions in mental, physical and social domains may all contribute to QoL, the weight of the different dimensions (in determining overall QoL) is likely to be very different between different patient populations. In Bernheim's view, multi-item questionnaires are seen to describe but not evaluate QoL – overall QoL can best be captured only via a global self-assessment.

To determine a clinically important difference

A further example of patient-based global health rating is in seeking to determine a 'minimal clinically important difference' or MCID for a HQoL measure. Hajiro & Nishimura (2002) observed how 'since there is no "gold standard" for measuring health status, health status measures may be compared or anchored to other clinical changes or results, which is called anchor-based interpretation'. The most commonly used anchor based interpretation is based on a patient global rating question. Patients are asked how they 'feel' about the effect of treatment or about their health.

Bottomley (2002) also referred to the approach to anchor changes seen in disease-specific questions to one regarding overall HQoL, such as, 'In general, how would you rate your quality of life?' Changes over time in answers to the global question could be compared with changes in a disease-specific questionnaire, with the changes in the disease-specific measures anchored to changes in overall health status.

For further discussion see Chapter 11 under 'Interpreting Quality of Life Scores for Individual Patients'.

To provide criterion measures in test development

An important use of patient global self-ratings is to provide a criterion to combine multiple dimensions when forming a HQoL instrument. The use of patient global ratings as criterion measures in test development is discussed later in this chapter ('Global Ratings as Criterion Measures in Test Development'). See also Chapter 4 under 'Criterion-related Validity'.

The responsiveness of global self-ratings

The empirical evidence is that a single item can be as good as a multi-item test (or at least a better choice in some circumstances).

Gardner et al (1998) conducted an empirical comparison of single item versus multiple item measurement scales in terms of ability to measure focus of attention at work. The evaluation entailed confirmatory factor analysis (CFA) statistical procedures, comparing the alternative scale forms on criteria of (a) convergent validity, (b) discriminant validity, and (c) degree of methods bias. The single-item was a 4 cm vertical line anchored by 'almost never' and 'almost all the time' and on which respondents indicated their response by placing a slash. The scales were scored by measuring the number of millimeters that respondents marked the line above 'almost never'. To create Likert-type items that corresponded to the vertical scales', the authors developed 4 items for each of 10 targets. Each item was scaled with a 5-point agree–disagree rating scale, resulting in a 40-item scale.

Gardner et al found that neither type of scale came out a clear 'winner'. Both scales converged as they should, diverged as they should, and showed statistically significant evidence of methods bias. It was concluded that the traditional multi-item measurement scales did not outperform the non-traditional single-item scales, and that where the use of a single-item was indicated, researchers could use them in the knowledge that they were acceptable.

The responsiveness of the single-item VAS has been reinforced by a number of other studies.

Sloan et al (1998) found that a single-item visual analogue index (the respondent placed an X in a long horizontal rectangle to indicate self-rated QoL over the past week) correlated strongly with the 22-item total score of the Functional Living Index-Cancer (FLIC), and was more responsive than the FLIC to changes in health of advanced cancer patients.

Hurny et al (1996) reported evaluation of a single-item linear analogue self-assessment scale for mood compared with a 28-item adjective checklist for emotional well-being with breast cancer in large multi-centre, multi-cultural trials. The results included the finding that both measures were responsive (out of 24 changes over time, 19 were in the expected direction for the linear analogue self-assessment scale, versus 17 for the adjective check list). The single-item was found to be more efficient for recurrence than the adjective checklist.

It was concluded that the single-item was a valid indicator of emotional well-being, and linear analogue self-assessment scales were supported as indicators of components of quality of life in cancer clinical trials.

Sloan et al (2002) conducted a comprehensive review of the evidence regarding the merits of single versus multi-item measures of QoL in cancer patients. They concluded that single items have the advantage of simplicity at the cost of detail, and multi-item indices have the advantage of providing a complete profile of QoL component constructs at the cost of increased burden and of asking potentially irrelevant questions. Moreover the two types of measure were able to be used together in a research study or a clinical setting.

As mentioned, a key issue is the degree to which a test item clearly targets the desired construct. The virtue of the single-item VAS is that the experimenter can specify the context and response scale precisely. The preamble framing the item can be precise, and the anchors to the VAS can be defined clearly and unambiguously to maximize its ability to measure the desired construct. While a single-item scale cannot convey *why* the magnitude is as estimated, the evidence is that it will provide a useful estimate of the size of patient-rated global HQoL.

VAS scales do have the disadvantage of being more onerous to score with the potential for clerical errors, and Donovan et al (1989) also noted that a question with a limited number of fixed response options tends to be easier to administer and score than an instrument employing continuous or VAS scales. However, Gardner et al suggested that single-item VAS scales also have potential advantages, as they:

- may produce a 'finer' measure than Likert scales
- are less time-consuming to develop than standard Likert-type items as fewer items need to be validated
- reduce the time required for respondents to complete the scales (as fewer items need to be completed)
- reduce the monotony inherent in questionnaires.

On asking patients to report only on effects due to the disease

In some tests, patients are asked to report only on effects due to the disease (this issue applies whether single or multiple items are being used). Ren & Kazis (1998) report creating a disease-specific physical functioning scale by adding the phrase 'because of your chronic lung disease', 'because of your chronic low back pain', or 'because of your knee osteoarthritis' to what were previously generic items.

While patients may at times be quite confident in their ability to report in this way, there can be no guarantee that they are correct in their identification of which effects are due to the targeted condition. Where the patient has multiple conditions (as many do), it would seem unwise indeed. In a research situation this issue can be dealt with through experimental design.

Most commonly it is better that the instrument lays out the domains most affecting HQoL; the clinician can then interpret the role of underlying pathology.

Cautions when using single-item tests

Single-item measures are frequently criticized for being unreliable and invalid. These arguments generally implicitly assume that the items are simple, e.g. a single line dichotomous item, or single word Likert response. Both Classical Test Theory (CTT) (e.g. Nunnally & Bernstein 1994) and Rasch/Item Response Theory (IRT) (e.g. Wright 1992) argue the merits of multi-item scales, although for somewhat different reasons (see Chs 6 and 8). As a result, nearly all measures of psychological attributes are multi-item measures.

In CTT, the argument is that any measure contains error, and random measurement error averages out when individual scores are summed. A remark often quoted in support of multi-item CTT tests is that 'other things being equal', a long test is more reliable than a short one (Nunnally 1978, p. 243). This same remark has also been criticized on the grounds that other things are never equal, as test items are selected, not randomly sampled (Gardner et al 1998, see also Wright 1992). Of course multi-item tests can only be superior if they assess the desired construct. Otherwise, a better-targeted single item is necessarily superior.

In contrast, the VAS items commonly used for gathering global HQoL measures are precisely defined, with a contextual preamble and anchors clearly and unambiguously described defining the construct to be measured. The previous section presented evidence that such single items can be as responsive to change as multi-item tests.

Certainly not all single item measures are suitable. The more complex tasks used by economists to elicit preferences (utilities) may not be appropriate. As mentioned earlier, Saigal et al (2001) found that 16% of patients were unable to comprehend the time tradeoff (TTO) task well enough to have utilities elicited. In this respect Kaplan et al (1993) observed that economists and psychologists differ in their preferred approaches to preference measurement, and that human information processors do poorly at integrating complex probability information. Such arguments support the use of simple rating scales. Giesler et al (1999) compared various methods of estimating utilities (measures of patient's preferences) with patients treated for advanced prostate cancer, assessing the rating scale, TTO, standard gamble and willingness to pay. They concluded that the rating scale performed best.

There are arguments that can be made against single items being *solely* relied upon for assessing patient-perceived HQoL. As discussed in Chapter 2 adaptation/response shift is an issue to be considered when interpreting test results. To identify and/or offset such effects, objective measures in addition to subjective measures are desirable.

A further criticism could be made by advocates of Rasch/IRT theory (see Ch. 8), namely that single item scales (such as the VAS) are necessarily non-interval. However, Rasch adherents would consider that Rasch scales can be converted to interval measures. Thomee et al (1995) applied Rasch analysis to VAS scores in assessing subjectively experienced pain experienced by women with patellofemoral pain syndrome (PFPS), and concluded that while patients with PFPS did not use the VAS as a linear scale over the full range, Rasch analysis of the VAS results gave a more detailed pain assessment.

With non-VAS scales, the number of response categories needs to be considered. Bond & Fox (2001) noted that rating scales should reflect careful consideration of the construct in question, and this should be conveyed with categories and labels that elicit unambiguous responses. In terms of the appropriate number of response categories for optimal measurement, Bond & Fox concluded that there was no definitive optimal number of response categories, and that the optimal number of response categories needed to be determined empirically every time a new rating scale was developed or used with a new population. Similarly empirical investigation is needed regarding labeling of response categories, use of anchors, etc.

GLOBAL RATINGS AS CRITERION MEASURES IN TEST DEVELOPMENT

Patient-reported global health-related quality of life can be a suitable criterion

A criterion is a variable that represents what the test is aiming to estimate, or that is very close to it. In assessing HQoL, the criterion can be a measure of patient-reported HQoL.

It would be difficult to make a case that someone other than the patient be accepted as the primary repository of information about the effects of any condition, particularly in the light of evidence that patients emphasize elements of their condition differently to others and generally differ from both doctors and the general public in their assessments of illness states.

As argued by Donovan et al (1989), if it is accepted that QoL is an individual's subjective sense of well-being, then it is necessarily the result of personal perception of circumstances, and any scale assessing QoL must be constructed using information from the patients themselves. Otherwise there is the risk of omitting information of central importance. At the very least, patient information should play a central role in the formation of any QoL instrument.

On the other hand, the evidence discussed earlier (Ch. 2) questions the wisdom of relying solely upon patient report, given the as yet poorly understood role and nature of adaptation. Healthcare givers, be they professional or voluntary, know to a greater or lesser extent the impact of factors related to health, while those intimate to the patient may know more fully of other factors and their interrelationships. Professional care givers can also have a broader knowledge of the comparative effects of different health states.

A related issue concerns who should complete tests that concern individual patient assessment. Donovan et al (1989) argued that such measures must be completed by patients, and not observers, for only the patient is fully aware of their own condition.

A number of instruments have been developed using assessments gathered from the public, and critics have asserted that this makes the instruments potentially irrelevant to patient populations.

Donovan et al (1989) concluded that a 1982 study by Irwin et al of the QoL of cancer survivors was of little value as it used an instrument that had little relevance in the context of cancer, the instrument being designed to measure QoL in healthy populations. Deyo & Patrick (1989) expressed concern regarding the fact that many health status questionnaires employ a 'weighting system' that assigns values to dysfunction based on the rankings of lay persons, noting that clinicians may be justifiably concerned that such standard weighting schemes may not reflect a particular patient's values. In this context, Kaplan & Anderson noted criticism of the Quality of Well-Being (QWB) scale for being developed on the basis of community rather than specific-population weights, and in part, defended this aspect by stating that Balaban et al (1986) found weights obtained with arthritis sufferers to be 'remarkably similar to those we obtained from members of the general population' (Kaplan & Anderson 1988).

Finally, it is desirable that criterions possess interval properties, are based on direct report (not other existing tests), and possess minimal error variance. None will be perfect, but the author's experience in health outcomes measurement is that it is generally possible to specify quite concretely what the test is aiming to assess (and indirectly maximize), and the most direct measure of this variable can be used beneficially.

Benefits of criterion measures

There are considerable advantages to having a strong criterion against which to assess and develop a test, as it hinders attempts to justify poorly formed or insensitive tests. The reason is that many tests are based on the sampling of what are alleged to be appropriate content areas, and certainly, content is central to the validity of multi-item HQoL measures. The test developers 'validate' their new measure by comparing its output to that of other measures, with relatively low correlations seen to confirm the merit of their instrument (if the correlations were high, they could be accused of merely reproducing an existing measure). Alternatively, the test might be applied to populations with very different levels of the construct (ambulation, depression, etc.), where even the most insensitive measure would be expected to reveal a difference. Content-oriented approaches can easily lead to flimsy tests. Unimpressive correlations can be justified on the grounds that 'there is no gold standard for tests of HQoL'.

It is interesting that this is not a recent phenomenon. Ebel (1961) observed that Toops (1944) stated some 50 years ago that 'the ease with which test developers can be induced to accept as criterion measures quantitative data [for test validation by correlation] having the slightest appearance of relevance to the trait being measured, is one of the scandals of psychometry'.

In the development of HQoL tests, there is an obvious strong criterion, i.e. some form of direct report from the patient of their self-assessed HQoL. However, this route is rarely taken. Ebrahim (1995) observed that in the assessment of reliability and validity of HQoL indicators 'content and construct validity are usually measured but the more important predictive validity is neglected'.

It is worthwhile to consider Toops again: 'Possibly as much time should be spent in devising the criterion as in constructing and perfecting the test. This important part of a research seldom receives half the time or attention it requires or deserves. If the criterion is slighted the time spent on the tests is, by so much, largely wasted' (Toops 1944; noted by Ebel 1961).

Box 5.1   Constructing an instrument with the aid of a VAS-based criterion: The Health Effects Scale (HES)

The Health Effects Scale (HES) was developed for ATSIC (The Australian 'Aboriginal and Torres Strait Islander Commission') to assess the relative severity of environmental conditions on health and so allow prioritization of the Aboriginal housing and infrastructure programme (O'Connor 1995).

The background was that the living conditions of many Australian Aborigines are comparable to the worst in the world, and health data revealed patterns of illness consistent with the effect of poor environmental conditions. A system for determining housing and infrastructure needs applied through points ratings and priorities was required. The instrument needed to:

i) provide a description of the 'environmental health' of a household (i.e. describe housing and infrastructure in health terms), and
ii) indicate which households were likely to be in the most health-threatening situation.

Due to the absence of adequate information in the literature, the HES was developed based on the judgment of individuals familiar with the effects of environmental conditions on health in Aboriginal or other developing communities. The group consisted of professionals in Aboriginal primary healthcare, environmental health, respiratory medicine, gastroenterology, microbiology, parasitology and health surveying. The process of development was to identify relevant environmental variables and form corresponding items/descriptors. The 'experts' then provided ratings on a VAS of 0 to 100 of the degree to which an environmental descriptor led to or was associated with adverse health effects (Zero was defined as signifying no adverse effect on health, and 100 as indicating that the environmental condition was severe, and 'likely to produce life-threatening or disabling disease or injury'). The resulting instrument was used to guide Aboriginal infrastructure development. The descriptors rated most severe are given in Figure 5.1.

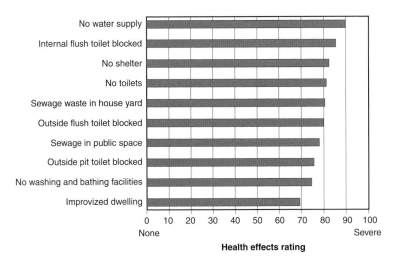

Figure 5.1 Top ten descriptors.

When dealing with tests based on multiple scales, a criterion also allows the development of an aggregated summary score. Without a criterion, the assignment of weightings to sub-scales becomes 'hit and miss' or arbitrary. Kaplan et al (1979) referred to this issue in arguing for the category rating task where a single global rating was given to case descriptions, allowing multiple dimensions of health to be considered jointly and simultaneously. They argued this was necessary if arbitrary rules for combining attributes into an overall rating were to be avoided.

Criterion measures (e.g. a measure of patient-reported global HQoL) also allow instruments to be improved, as variability that is not accounted for by the instrument under development may indicate important domains that have been neglected.

SUMMARY

Single item scales

- Context effects can be minimized by the use of rating scales where there has been careful definition of the the end-points and the continuum along which states are to be rated. Clearly labelled visual analogue rating scales are well supported.

- Terms should be operationalized where possible, e.g. terms such as 'frequently', 'seldom', or 'hardly ever'; thus 'hardly ever' can become 'once a month or less', etc.
- Complex tasks should be avoided so as to focus on the primary aspect of interest, i.e. perception/experience of a health state.
- The nature of the item frame is very important: testees respond in different ways when presented with essentially the same information but different references and formats.

Patient global self-ratings

Estimate overall HQoL:
- To evaluate diverse outcomes after treatment.
- To appraise validity of a summated multi-component score.

Capture the individual's unique self-report:
- Some multi-item questionnaires describe aspects of a patient's experience but do not allow a personalized self-assessment.

Determine a clinically important difference:
- The most commonly used anchor to determine a clinically important difference in test score is patients' global rating of how they 'feel' about the effect of treatment or about their health (also see Ch. 11 under 'Interpreting Quality of Life Scores for Individual Patients').

Provide criterion measures in test development:
- to weight and combine multiple dimensions.

Global self-ratings can be responsive

There is evidence that a single-item VAS can be as good or better than multi-item tests in assessing responsiveness in cancer patients. They also have the potential advantages of:
- Being less time-consuming to develop than Likert-type items as fewer items need to be validated.
- Reducing the time required for respondents to complete the scales (fewer items need to be completed).

Cautions when using single-item tests

- Single-item measures can be less reliable and valid – if they are brief and poorly formed, have inadequate framing, or entail complex tasks.

- Several items may be desirable if assessing patient-perceived HQoL – to gather both objective and subjective estimates where adaptation is a concern.
- Single-item scales such as the VAS may be non-interval, but could be converted to interval measures using the Rasch model.
- Can be unsuitable if they lack sufficient response labels.

Global ratings as criterion measures in test development

The benefits of a criterion measure include:

- Frustrating the development of poor tests, such as tests justified based on comparisons with existing tests where low correlations are seen as justified.
- Facilitating the development of an overall rating by providing a way of combining and weighting sub-scales, so avoiding arbitrary combination rules.
- Providing a means of improving existing instruments by revealing the need for additional or improved content (to explain variability not accounted for).

FURTHER POINTS

- While a single item will provide relatively little information, it can be phrased in such a way as to target the issue of primary interest. If HQoL is identified with patient self-report, then a simple approach is to gather a global self-assessment from the patient and use this as a criterion measure in test development. Cancer studies have found global reports using VAS scales to exhibit high responsiveness.
- The following guidelines are suggested concerning the role of global self-assessment in developing a multi-item HQoL test:
  - Recognize that simple patient report may not provide an unblemished criterion measure of HQoL, but it is still the best simple direct measure of patient health status from the patient's perspective, and an item can be formed to precisely target the test construct.
  - In developing the test, separate the elements involved in the development of a test measure, from the elements of the

developed test. A single-item measure of self-reported global health might play a central role during test development, but a different role in the final instrument (expectancies, demand characteristics, and adaptation effects, may lead to changes in self-assessment which are unrelated to specific changes in the illness state or medical treatment).

- Consider comprehensively assessing the variables that affect the patients HQoL via individual sub-scales, and use the single-item criterion measure to develop a weighting system to assess their relative importance.

- Include a global self-report item as a general catch-all in the final measurement instrument (to detect any key influence that might otherwise be overlooked).

Classical approaches to test development

AIMS OF CHAPTER

• To describe the theoretical basis underlying the most common multi-item scale, namely the sum-scale based on Classical Test Theory (CTT), and describe the Likert scale

• To introduce the notion of reliability, statistics used to assess reliability, and describe factors that influence reliability estimates

• To introduce the standard error of measurement (SEM) and its role in setting confidence intervals for test scores

• To introduce alternative approaches to scale building, by Thurstone and by Guttman

THE SUM SCALE APPROACH OF CLASSICAL TEST THEORY (CTT)

Classical approaches define the strength of the attribute (or ability) in terms of the observed score. This is in contrast to modern test theory or 'latent trait theory', which estimates the strength of the attribute in terms of the underlying trait (the 'true score' of Classical Test Theory (CTT)).

CTT is a 'linear, summative or centroid model' where the total score summarizes all the important information about the attribute (Nunnally & Bernstein 1994).

True score and error

CTT makes the assumption that an observed test or item score can be decomposed into two parts: a 'true' score representing the value of the attribute or construct, the value of which no one really knows, and an 'error' score, i.e.:

'observed score' = 'true score' + random error

Sum-scale tests aim to identify and gather results from a large number of items. Because the error term is by definition random, the more items that are gathered and averaged, the more likely that the average will approach an accurate estimate of true score, i.e. the amount of attribute, as the summed errors will approach zero.

According to Nunnally & Bernstein (1994), the CTT model makes no assumptions about the distribution of scores, is tolerant of guessing and/or carelessness, is 'simple, makes sense, and works well in practice'.

While CTT has been the dominant theoretical model underlying health outcomes tests, it is currently under challenge from Rasch analysis/Item Response Theory (IRT) (see Ch. 8).

Item difficulty and item discrimination

Item difficulty in CTT is the overall proportion of correct response (or report indicating more of the attribute) to a particular item for a group of testees, often referred to as the 'p' value of the item (the index of item difficulty).

In CTT, item parameters such as item difficulty (and item discrimination) are a property of the group that responded to them, not the item. This is unlike item difficulty as defined under IRT, where it has a consistent meaning that is independent of the group used to obtain its value (Baker 2001).

Item discrimination is the capacity of an item to discriminate between high and low ability testees in the behaviour or attribute that the test is designed to measure. A discriminating item is more likely to be endorsed by a person who has a high total score than by someone with a low total score, i.e. the item discriminates between those who score high and hence are supposed to have more of the trait, and those who score low.

Item discrimination can be indicated by the degree to which the score on the item correlates with the total test score. This is often expressed statistically as the Pearson's Product Moment Correlation coefficient between scores on the item and scores on the total test; for dichotomous items (e.g. items with response options such as 'yes' and 'no') the estimate is often made via the point-biserial correlation coefficient.

Items with low item-total correlations are generally deleted to maximize unidimensionality, homogeneity, and reliability. Items with low correlations (e.g. lower than 0.25) add little meaningful variance to the total test score, lower the reliability of the test, and increase the likelihood that differences in total scores may be due to chance. Note that difficulty and discrimination are not independent. If all testees either pass or fail an item, the item does not discriminate. Item discrimination is maximized when half of the test takers answer an item in the way indicating more of the attribute, i.e. when $p = 0.50$ (e.g. Zurawski 1998).

While there are theoretical weaknesses in CTT, such as non-independence of item and person statistics (see 'The Rasch Model', Ch. 8), most of these aspects have been handled through ad hoc empirical procedures (Fan 1998), e.g. test equating via equipercentile equating, or item-invariant measurement via Thurstone's Absolute Scaling (see the following).

Thurstone Absolute Scaling

There can be a need to form a scale made up of items scored by different subject groups. A solution is to use a fixed, standard reference group to define the scale units and origin and to then convert all subsequent scores to that scale via common anchor or linkage items included in the tests administered to each sample. A different set of linkage items can be shared by different pairs of

---

Box 6.1 An example of a Likert scale item from the Asthma Medication Adherence Questionnaire (AMAQ) (O'Connor et al 2000)

Please indicate the extent to which the following statements reflect your views/experience of your scheduled medication over the last three months. (Please tick one box only for each statement.)
Overall, my scheduled medication:

	Strongly disagree	Disagree	Neither agree nor disagree	Agree	Strongly agree
a. Makes me feel better			✓		

---

groups, but with each sample linked to the others to form a chain extending to the reference group. The statistical procedure, known as absolute scaling, was developed by Thurstone and has been widely applied in test development (see Anastasi 1990, Nunnally & Bernstein 1994, Anastasi & Urbina 1997).

The Likert scale: common item type used in Classical Test Theory tests

One of the most common types of item used in CTT-based tests is the Likert scale. Likert scales consist of an item stem and a series of statements, one of which is selected to convey a graded response. Response statements are typically scored with a 1 to 5 or 1 to 7 format ('Strongly disagree' = 1, 'Disagree' = 2, 'Neither agree nor disagree' = 3, etc.).

An example of a Likert scale item is shown in Box 6.1.

Likert items are typically scored as if all items are of equal value and the response alternatives have interval properties.

THE ROLE OF 'RELIABILITY' IN CLASSICAL TEST THEORY

As put by Anastasi (1990), *measures of test reliability estimate the proportion of test variability that is due to error variance*, where error variance is change in scores due to anything other than the characteristic of interest.

Reliability inherently attenuates the maximum possible magnitude of relationships between variables. All else being constant, poor score reliability will reduce the power of statistical significance tests.

The need to minimize error variance is the reason why psychological tests typically specify all aspects of the test environment, i.e. instructions, time limits, mode of subject-tester interaction, etc., the aim being to eliminate or control extraneous sources of variance that would otherwise affect test results.

There are many approaches to estimating reliability, each of which generates a different coefficient. For example, one can compare different raters with the same subjects (inter-rater), same subjects separated by a short time interval (test-retest), items with each other or the total (internal consistency), different forms of the test (parallel forms), and so on.

The basic measure of test reliability or reliability coefficient is the *correlation coefficient*, which indicates the consistency between two independently derived sets of scores. The most common of these is Pearson's Product Moment Correlation. Significance tests can determine the probability of the observed correlation occurring by chance alone.

The reliability of a test's scores should always be *reported and considered in result interpretation*, in all forms applicable, i.e. internal consistency reliability, test-retest reliability, inter-rater reliability, etc. Moreover, reliability should be reported for scores in the study, not estimates from prior studies or test manuals, as the same measure when administered to more or less homogeneous subjects will yield scores with differing reliability. Henson (2001) points out that it is more appropriate to speak of the reliability of 'test scores' or the 'measurement' than of the 'test'.

Pearson's Product Moment Correlation **compares scores of two variables in terms of the amount of deviation (paired) scores display above or below the respective group mean scores. It determines the standard scores for all scores in each variable, and calculates the product of the paired scores, the correlation coefficient being the mean of these products.**

Measures of internal consistency

Internal consistency estimates are among the most common forms of reliability coefficients because they are readily calculated from a single administration of a test. It is nearly impossible to see a scale development paper that has not used Cronbach's Alpha (Streiner & Norman 1996, Henson 2001).

In CTT the test is treated as if it is made up of a random sampling of all possible items that could be in the test. If so, the items should be highly interrelated because they assess the same construct of interest (e.g. health-related quality of life [HQoL] self-esteem, etc.). If items are highly correlated, it is theoretically assumed that the construct of interest has been measured to some degree of consistency, i.e. the scores are reliable (Henson 2001).

Cronbach's Alpha

The most common procedure for finding inter-item consistency is Cronbach's Alpha, where:

$$\alpha = [n/(n-1)] \times [1 - (\Sigma\sigma_i^2/\sigma_T^2)]$$

(n = the number of items, σ_i is the standard deviation for each item, and σ_T is the standard deviation of the total score).

The Kuder-Richardson formula 20 (KR-20) reliability coefficient takes a similar approach (e.g. see Crocker & Algina 1986, Streiner & Norman 1996), but the KR-20 works only when test items are dichotomously scored (e.g. 0 and 1) while Cronbach's Alpha (also known as Coefficient alpha or α) can be used both with dichotomously scored items and measures using multiple response categories, such as Likert scale data. For an illustration of the way Cronbach's Alpha may be applied, see StatSoft (1999).

Streiner & Norman (1996) note that the implication is usually made that the higher the coefficient, the better. However, there are problems in uncritically accepting high values of Alpha:

Firstly, a high Alpha does not simply reflect high internal consistency. Alpha is dependent not only on the magnitude of the correlations among the items, but also on the number of items in the scale. Alpha can be increased simply by increasing the number of items, even though the average correlation remains the same. The result of this is that a list of items may actually consist of, say, two distinct sets of items measuring two distinct constructs. Alpha could be high because of the large number of items, despite the fact that it is tapping two different attributes.

The opposite problem is that if Alpha is too high, it may suggest too high a level of item redundancy (i.e. items asking the same question in slightly different ways). This may indicate that the scale as a whole is too narrow in its scope to have much validity. A highly relevant question then is whether the construct that the test is trying to predict is itself relatively homogeneous or heterogeneous. 'A single homogeneous test is obviously not an adequate predictor of a highly heterogeneous criterion' (Anastasi 1990, p. 123).

How large does internal consistency need to be?

The size of an internal consistency estimate required varies depending on the purposes of the research and uses of the scores. Aaronson et al (2002) describe commonly accepted minimal standards for reliability coefficients as 0.70 for group comparisons and 0.90–0.95 for individual comparisons (see also Nunnally & Bernstein 1994). In contrast, Streiner & Norman (1996) maintain that measures of internal consistency should always be interpreted with great caution.

As internal consistency estimates apply to test items assumed to represent a single underlying construct, tests consisting of scales measuring different constructs require separate internal consistency estimates for each scale.

Test-retest or measure of stability/reproducibility

The most obvious means for estimating the reliability of a test is through re-presenting the identical test on a later occasion. The correlation coefficient for a test-retest procedure is termed the *coefficient of stability*. The Pearson's Product Moment Correlation formula can be used.

Crocker & Algina (1986) state that few if any standards exist for judging the minimally acceptable value for a coefficient of stability, but that commercially published, individually administered aptitude tests are amongst the highest. Subsets of the Weschler Adult Intelligence Scale (WAIS) have coefficients in the 0.70s, 0.80s, and low 0.90s. Personality, interest or attitude measures are often lower than these, but Crocker & Algina propose that a well constructed test should still have test-retest coefficients in the 0.80s.

For tests used to make a decision about individuals, Streiner & Norman (1996) cite possible acceptable reliability values as 0.85 (citing Kelley 1927) to 0.94 (citing Weiner & Stewart 1984). They also note that a test used for individual judgment should be more reliable than one used for group decisions or research purposes, given that research will draw conclusions from a mean score averaged across many individuals, and the sample size will serve to reduce the error of measurement in comparison to group differences. A sample of 1000 can tolerate a much less reliable instrument than a sample of 10, so that the acceptable reliability is dependent on the sample size used in the research (elsewhere Streiner & Norman suggest stability measures greater than 0.5 could suffice under some conditions).

Although apparently simple and straightforward, and recommended by Streiner & Norman on the grounds that they allow the effects of a number of sources of error to be assessed, these tests can be hard to interpret. Basically the two testings cannot be considered as independent, due to practice and/or recall, and while the longer the interval between test and retest is, the less is the risk of memory effects, and the greater is the risk of intervening events causing respondents to change their views. Hence the obtaining of a low coefficient may mean either the test is an unreliable measure of the construct, or the construct has changed in magnitude. Alternatively, a high coefficient may reflect a change in the testee's behaviour since the first administration, and reflect effects of memory, practice, learning, sensitization etc. In assessing a test-retest correlation, it is hard to decide if it has been inflated (due to memory effects), or deflated (due to change in the attribute being assessed).

(For consideration of other reliability forms, e.g. measure of equivalence, see Anastasi & Urbina 1997.)

Factors that affect reliability coefficients

Characteristics of the subjects: variation in the behaviour, and ability to perform the measurement task

An important factor influencing the size of a reliability coefficient is the range of individual differences in the group, or *subject* (as opposed to item) *homogeneity*.

If members of the test group are similar with respect to the trait being measured, then the reliability coefficient will be much lower than if they varied markedly regarding the trait, because the random error variance will tend to be constant for the two groups (if of equal size), while 'true' score variance will be much less and hence account for a much smaller proportion of the observed score variance. In other words a test is not reliable or unreliable – reliability is a property of the scores on a test for a particular group of subjects. A consequence of this is that to compare tests, it is essential to determine whether reported reliability estimates were based on samples similar in composition.

A further factor influencing the size of the reliability coefficient is the *general ability level of the group in test-taking per se*. For example, if the subjects are confused or pressured by the demands of the task, then there is likely to be increased error variance, and hence reduced test reliability. On the other hand, it may be difficult to justify eliminating such subjects, particularly if they represent a particular group, e.g. patients or patients' relatives as opposed to health professionals – patients and their relatives may possess less formal education and be relatively unfamiliar with formal testing procedures, but at the same time possess relevant and valuable knowledge of health status variables and their effects. Eliminating such subjects because they fail to master the task is likely to reduce the test's validity.

Examiner variance as a source of error, i.e. variation in test scores as a product of experimenter/examiner factors should also be considered, and if necessary, controlled for (Anastasi 1990, p. 125).

Test items: test length and homogeneity

As already noted, test length affects both true score variance and observed score variance. Longer tests have greater test reliability than shorter tests composed of similar items (errors of measurement due to content sampling are reduced).

The Spearman-Brown prophecy formula can be used to estimate the effects on reliability of increasing or decreasing test size. As pointed out by Moser & Kalton (1979, p. 355), if the correlation between two items is 0.5, and both items were used in the test, the Spearman-Brown formula calculates their reliability at 0.67. If further items all inter-correlated 0.5 were added, the reliability would increase further. The higher the inter-correlation between items, the less the number needed to reach a given level of reliability. Thus only 4 items inter-correlated at 0.7 are needed to reach a *stepped-up reliability* or $r_w = 0.9$, but 9 items are needed if they were inter-correlated at 0.5.

In measuring attributes, the set of items may not intercorrelate highly, and to attain an adequate level of reliability, multiple items are needed: the higher the intercorrelation between items, i.e. the greater the item homogeneity, the less items are needed (Moser & Kalton 1979). On the other hand, item homogeneity may only be obtained by restricting the breadth of the scale, and this may have a direct effect on reducing validity (see below and Ch. 4 under 'The Role of Multiple Regression in HQoL Measurement').

Cautions with reliability coefficients

Each of the multiple forms of reliability identifies and quantifies only one source of error variance which are separate and cumulative (internal consistency, test-retest, inter-rater, etc.). Obtaining an $\alpha = 0.90$ does not mean this is the overall reliability for the scores, as further measurement error could be found in a test-retest or inter-rater coefficient, which explains different sources of error (Henson 2001; also Streiner & Norman 1996).

Much care needs to be taken when interpreting reliability coefficients, for they are relevant only to the group of subjects upon which the test was developed. Analogously, when comparing the reliability of tests, the reliability estimates need to have been based on similar subjects (i.e. the size of a reliability coefficient will tend to be proportional to the variability between subjects).

As described, high test reliability may come at a cost. Test reliability is directly related to item homogeneity, but item homogeneity is increased by restricting the breadth of the scale. When a test is assessing a highly heterogeneous construct such as HQoL, there can be a tradeoff between test reliability and test validity. A high reliability coefficient indicates there is consistency in a testee's scores; it does not ensure that the inference to be drawn for the test is correct. Nonetheless, reliability is a necessary (but not sufficient) condition for validity, and low reliability will limit validity.

> **When examining reliability coefficients, healthy scepticism is recommended regarding what is purported to be demonstrated, combined with a close examination of the item and subject conditions.**

The Standard Error of Measurement: setting confidence intervals and assessing test score differences

Error in the measurement process can be thought of as any factor entering into the process that is not directly relevant to whatever it is that is being measured. This may be a poorly reproduced test form (hard to read), excessive noise in the testing environment, items assessing factors other than that under examination, the subject's health if it is affecting completing the questionnaire, etc. Any number of factors other than the construct being tested can enter into the process of measuring the attitude/trait/ability. This is why it is important to reduce error in a testing situation to the extent that it is possible. However, one can never entirely eliminate error. The best one can do is estimate how much error entered into a particular test score and then intelligently interpret the score with that information (Cohen & Swerdlick 1999, pp. 23, 166). Note that Generalisability Theory is particularly concerned with the issue of attributing error to its various sources (see Streiner & Norman 1996).

A statistic used to estimate or infer how far *observed* scores deviate from *true* scores is the *standard error of measurement* (SEM).

In the case of a test, the SEM would be equal to the standard deviation of the observed test results scores. In practice, few developers of tests designed for use on a widespread basis would investigate the magnitude of error with respect to a single test taker; more typically, an average SEM is calculated for a sample of the population on which the test is designed for use.

Determining confidence intervals for a test score

The reliability coefficient helps the test developer build an adequate measuring instrument and it helps the test user select a suitable test. However, an obtained test score represents one point in the distribution of scores the test-taker could have obtained, and the test user has no way of knowing the test-taker's true score. The reliability coefficient can be employed in the formula for the SEM to describe the amount of error in a test or a measure. If the standard deviation for the distribution of test scores is known or can be calculated, the SEM can be determined.

The SEM may be considered as the average standard deviation of examinees' individual error distributions for a large number of repeated testings, and allows the establishment of a confidence interval, a range or band of test scores that is likely to contain the true score.

Thus the true score is likely to lie within ±2 SEMs (approx.) of the observed score (e.g. see Anastasi 1990, Crocker & Algina 1986). The standard error of measurement (abbreviated to SEM, SEm, or σ_{meas}) is also known as the *standard error of a score*, and is defined in terms of the standard deviation at baseline (σ) and the reliability of the HQoL measure (R) where:

$$\sigma_{meas} = \sigma\sqrt{1 - R}$$

(see Anastsi & Urbina 1997, Wyrwich & Wolinsky 2000)

If the standard deviation of a test is held constant, as R increases, the SEM decreases. The SEM, and the reliability coefficient, are alternative ways of expressing test reliability. The reliability coefficient is best for comparing the reliability of different tests, and the SEM is recommended for the interpretation of individual scores. Anastasi (1990) recommends that when the score for a test is reported, an indication of its expected error should be provided.

Streiner & Norman (1996, p. 114) argue that the measure of reliability to be used in calculating SEM is probably most defensibly one based on test-retest, as measures of internal consistency (such as Cronbach Alpha) they are based on performance observed in a single sitting and cannot take account of the many sources of variance which occur from day to day or between observers.

Determining whether or not test scores (on the same test) are different

The interpretation of score differences should be made via measures of the standard error of score differences (e.g. see Anastasi 1990). The SEM cannot be used to compare scores, as the standard error of the difference between two scores will be larger than the SEM for either score alone, given that it is affected by measurement error in *both* scores. The formula for the standard error of the difference between two scores is:

$$\sigma_{diff} = \sqrt{(\sigma^2_{meas\ 1} + \sigma^2_{meas\ 2})}$$

where σ_{diff} is the standard error of the difference between two scores, $\sigma_{meas\,1}^2$ is the squared SEM for test 1, and $\sigma_{meas\,2}^2$ is the squared SEM for test 2. If reliability coefficients are substituted for the SEM of the separate scores, the formula becomes:

$$\sigma_{diff} = \sigma\sqrt{(2 - R_1 - R_2)}$$

where R_1 is the reliability coefficient of test 1, R_2 is the reliability coefficient of test 2, and σ is the standard deviation (both tests having the same standard deviation).

The value obtained when the standard error of the difference is calculated is used in much the same way as the standard error of the mean. To be 95% confident that the two scores are different, they would need to be separated by 1.96 standard errors of the difference. A separation of only one standard error of the difference would give 68% confidence that the two scores are different.

LIMITATIONS OF CLASSICAL TEST THEORY

CTT is focused on the formation of individual unidimensional scales (as are IRT/Rasch models). This reflects its origins in education and psychology where the dominant concern had been to assess unidimensional attributes such as maths competence, anxiety, etc.

In contrast, health outcomes measures may be seeking to estimate an outcome as complex as the effects of a treatment for HIV/AIDS. Berzon et al (1997) reported nine dimensions relevant to assessing the effects of early HIV disease, including sexual functioning, worries regarding disclosure of disease status, cognitive functioning and ability to perform basic activities of daily living. Each of these may be best considered as a unidimensional scale (although some may need to be further divided and others better amalgamated).

While a series of unidimensional scales may play a key role in monitoring areas of vital importance to patients, there is still a need for a measure of the relative and combined effect of the dimensions, both to indicate their relative importance and to determine the extent to which changes in the overall state represent an improvement in health (or a lesser decline).

This 'problem' is shared with Rasch/IRT models (see Ch. 8 under 'Rasch and Tests Based on Multiple Dimensions'), and there are ways to deal with it. One option is to develop a further superordinate, unidimensional scale, assuming that was possible. An alternative is an index which assesses and incorporates each dimension based on its ability to predict a criterion (see Ch. 5 under 'Global Ratings as Criterion Measures in Test Development' and Ch. 7 under 'Developing a Method for Combining Sub-test Scores').

However, there is a further problem, namely that the CTT approach is based on observed scores that can be criticized as having ordinal properties only and that do not provide interval measures. Many IRT/Rasch advocates consider this criticism damning. Chapter 8 describes how Rasch/IRT models deal with the issue.

Another problem is that CTT can act as if items have equal amounts of the attribute. This can seem very unsatisfactory in the health setting (an ambulation scale should treat the item 'able to run' as indicating more ability than the item 'able to stand').

Models that recognize item differences and pursue interval measures are those of Thurstone and Guttman. These are discussed in the following sections.

THURSTONE'S METHODS

The methods of Thurstone attempt to determine the quantitative values of individual items in terms of the continuum of the attribute being assessed, i.e. to determine the scale-values of items.

Thurstone developed both direct/subjective, and indirect/discriminant models (Nunnally & Bernstein 1994).

Direct model: Thurstone's Method of Equal-appearing Intervals

The Method of Equal-appearing Intervals is a direct model where items are rated directly by the subject (and most commonly by a group of subjects), the rating or average forming the scale value of the item.

A large set of statements assumed to measure a single construct are first formed. Expert judges then rate each statement on a 1 to 11 scale in terms of how much each statement indicates the quantity being assessed (a clear description of the concept to be measured and the scoring task is essential so the experts providing the scores have a clear idea of what they are to estimate).

For example, to develop a scale for measuring degree of dysphagia, six speech therapists might be asked to rate a series of items, where scores are to reflect the degree to which the item indicates 'difficulty in transferring food from the mouth to the stomach'. With an 11 point scale, '1' might be 'no problem at all in transferring food to the stomach', and '11' 'no ability to transfer food from mouth to stomach'. Items with excessive variability (low agreement) between judges would be either excluded, or rephrased and re-rated, and the average values across judges calculated to form the scale values of each item.

Examples of use

The Method of Equal-appearing Intervals was employed in the formation of the Sickness Impact Profile (SIP) (Bergner et al 1976a, 1976b, 1981; for a comprehensive description see Ch. 9).

Keller et al (1998b) used a variation of the Thurstone method of equal appearing intervals to evaluate the response labels used in the SF-36. Judges from different countries marked a point on a 10 cm line representing the magnitude of each response label relative to anchors of 'poor' and 'excellent'. Ratings were evaluated to determine the ordinal consistency of response choice labels, and the degree to which differences were equal interval, etc. Desselle et al (2002) reported using a method of equal-appearing intervals to create a performance appraisal template for pharmacy technicians.

Indirect model: Thurstone's Law of Comparative Judgement and the Method of Paired Comparisons

A probabilistic indirect method for developing interval scales is Thurstone's Law of Comparative Judgement, which leads directly to modern indirect models such as the Rasch model (both are 'representational models': see Ch. 8 under 'Should Measures of Psychological Attributes Have Interval Properties').

While applying the Method of Paired Comparisons is very demanding of resources and, therefore, rarely adopted, it is worth considering in some detail as it aids understanding of the increasingly popular Rasch model.

The Law of Comparative Judgement entails the following (derived from the characterization provided by Nunnally & Bernstein 1994, pp. 56–64):

- For a specified attribute, a given stimulus is assumed to yield a set of varying responses (e.g. if measuring 'depression', the degree of agreement with the statement 'I often feel down' will be reflected in the probability of 'agree' versus 'disagree').
- The variation in response to any stimulus is assumed to be normally distributed, and the mean of the responses to the stimulus is the best estimate of the scale value of that stimulus.
- The mean values of the sets of responses to stimuli correlate with intensity of the attribute on an interval scale.
- For stimuli sufficiently adjacent on the attribute continuum, the response distributions will overlap.

The Method of Paired Comparisons uses the degree to which the responses to two stimuli overlap to calculate the distance apart of stimuli on the hypothesized underlying scale of the attribute. A degree of observed overlap is essential, otherwise the location of the stimulus on the underlying interval attribute scale cannot be determined. (IRT/Rasch models similarly require 'response overlap' to determine location on the attribute continuum; see Ch. 8 under 'The Rasch Model'.)

In essence, the method is to present pairs of stimuli, say S1 and S2, for judgement in terms of which signifies the greater amount of the attribute. The proportion of times S1 is judged greater than S2 is determined, and the proportion converted into a corresponding number of standard deviation units from a table of the normal distribution to yield the difference (as the individual sets of responses to S1 and S2 are assumed to be normally distributed, the distribution of their difference will also be normally distributed). By this method, intervals are computed for all pairs of stimuli. For further discussion and explanation see Nunnally & Bernstein (1994).

While greatly time consuming (with 50 items, each judge would need to make 1225 judgements) and relatively complex, the procedure produces an interval scale.

The scale formed is still dependent upon the sample used in its formation, a deficiency claimed to be avoided when scales are formed using the Rasch model. The Rasch and IRT models do not use the cumulative normal distribution, as did Thurstone, but the ogival logistic distribution (similar but more convenient mathematically).

GUTTMAN'S 'DETERMINISTIC' MODEL

Guttman scales also allocate scale values to items. In a Guttman scale, items are ordered along a continuum of attribute strength, so that when it is judged that an attribute described by an item is achieved, all items signifying lesser attribute strength are also achieved. Again, the purpose of Guttman scaling is to establish a one-dimensional continuum.

The essential procedure in the development of the scale is to identify a set of items that fall into an ordered sequence in terms of attribute strength. The individual items can then be rated by expert judges to determine their scale values, and items then selected based on low variability across judges and desired spread across the scale.

A variant of a Guttman scale is given below in Box 6.2. The scale is to be completed by a medical officer after a comprehensive examination of the patient. The task is to identify the item-task most closely describing the subject's ability.

The item response options that form Guttman scales have several potential advantages over the response options in Likert scales. These include:

- Can employ multiple graded options which together clearly define the area being assessed and so reduce ambiguity (and hence reduce error).
- The individual item-options can be extensively described and operationalized, and hence further reduce misunderstanding and error.

Box 6.2 A variant of a Guttman scale from the Work Ability Tables (O'Connor et al 1996)

Table 6: Ability to manipulate objects for work, over the next two years.
   This Table measures the impact of the applicant's impairment upon their ability to manipulate everyday and work objects.

   0   While may experience some discomfort, able to manipulate objects freely.
  30   Some reduction in dexterity and/or speed of manipulation of objects as a result of impairment(s), e.g. difficulty smoothly placing key in lock, teaspoon of sugar in coffee, but able to turn door handles, manipulate money, write, use a keyboard, use hand tools, etc.
  75   Substantially diminished dexterity and/or speed of manipulation as a result of impairment(s), unable to turn door handles and/or manipulate money, write, use a keyboard, use hand tools, etc.

- Every item-option can have a different score: hence equal differences between item response options are not assumed.

Guttman scaling is a deterministic model; it assumes there is no error. Andrich (1982) notes that realization of a Guttman scale is enhanced if items have a large spread in difficulty, and if no two items are close together on the scale. It helps also if the range of abilities of individuals is relatively large, covering the wide range of item difficulties.

The Guttman scale is a basic link to modern test theory, but where the deterministic step function has been replaced with a probabilistic ogive (Nunnally & Bernstein 1994, see also Andrich 1982, Wright 1999). Thus the Rasch model is a probabilistic counterpart of the Guttman scale: if item difficulties are spread greatly, then responses generated according to the Rasch model will reveal a Guttman pattern (Andrich 1982). As described by Nunnally & Bernstein (1994), ogival models make good intuitive sense as they assume uncertainty as opposed to the perfect discrimination in a Guttman scale. IRT/Rasch models are discussed in Chapter 8.

SUMMARY

The sum scale approach

- Classical approaches define the strength of the attribute (or ability) in terms of the observed score, in contrast to modern test theory which estimates the strength of the attribute in terms of the underlying, latent trait.
- CTT assumes that an observed test or item score can be decomposed into a 'true' score representing the value of the attribute, and an 'error' score. 'Observed score' = 'true score' + random error.
- Sum-scale tests aim to identify and gather results from a large number of items. Because the error term is by definition random, the more items that are averaged, the more the average approaches the amount of the attribute, as the summed errors will approach zero.
- Item difficulty in CTT is the overall proportion of correct response (or report indicating more of the attribute) to a

particular item for a group of testees, often referred to as the 'p' value of the item (the index of item difficulty).
- Item discrimination is the capacity of an item to discriminate between high and low ability testees in the behaviour or attribute that the test is designed to measure.

The role of 'reliability' in Classical Test Theory

- Test reliability indicates the proportion of test variability due to error variance.
- Low reliability reduces the magnitude of relationships between variables.
- Tests of reliability include intra-observer, inter-observer, test-retest, and internal consistency.
- The basic measure of test reliability is the correlation coefficient, and the most common is Pearson's Product Moment Correlation.
- The reliability of a test's scores should always be reported and considered in all forms applicable.

Internal consistency reliability:

- Internal consistency estimates are common because they can be calculated from a single administration of a test.
- If items are highly correlated, it is theoretically assumed that the construct of interest has been measured to some degree of consistency, i.e. the scores are reliable.

Cronbach's Alpha:

- A high Alpha is dependent on the number of items in the scale as well as high internal consistency; Alpha could be high because of the large number of items while tapping two different attributes.
- If Alpha is too high it may suggest too high a level of item redundancy (i.e. items asking the same question in slightly different ways). This may indicate that the scale as a whole is too narrow in its scope to have much validity.
- Values of Alpha suggested for group comparisons are 0.7 and 0.90–0.95 for individual comparisons.
- For tests consisting of scales measuring different constructs, separate internal consistency estimates need to be made for each scale.

Test-retest reliability:

- The most obvious means for estimating the reliability of a test is through representing the identical test on a later occasion. The correlation coefficient for a test-retest procedure is termed the coefficient of stability, and again the Pearson's Product Moment Correlation formula can be used.
- For tests used to make a decision about individuals, Streiner & Norman (1996) cite possible acceptable reliability values as 0.85 to 0.94, and suggest stability measures greater than 0.5 could suffice under some conditions.
- Test-retest measures can be hard to interpret. While the longer the interval is between test and retest the less is the risk of memory effects, the greater is the risk of intervening events causing respondents to change their views.

Factors that affect reliability coefficients
Subjects:

- Variability in the subjects in the trait being assessed. A test is not reliable or unreliable – reliability is a property of the scores on a test for a particular group of subjects. The greater the variability in the subjects in the trait being assessed, the higher the reliability coefficient will be.
- High test-taking ability. If the subjects are confused or pressured by the demands of the task, then there is likely to be increased error variance, and hence reduced test reliability.
- Low examiner variance, i.e. little variation in test scores as a product of experimenter/examiner factors.

Test items:

- Longer tests have greater test reliability than shorter tests composed of similar items as errors of measurement due to content sampling are reduced.
- Item homogeneity – the higher the intercorrelation between items, i.e. the greater the item homogeneity, the less items are needed.

Cautions with reliability coefficients:

- Each of the multiple forms of reliability identifies and quantifies only one source of error variance that is separate and cumulative (internal consistency, test-retest, inter-rater, etc.).

- Reliability coefficients apply only to the group upon which the test was developed.
- Test reliability is directly related to item homogeneity, but there can be a tradeoff between test reliability and test validity.

The standard error of measurement
The SEM is used to:

- Estimate how far observed scores deviate from true scores.
- Determine confidence intervals for a test score.
- Determine whether test scores (on the same test) are different.

Limitations of Classical Test Theory

- CTT is focused on the formation of individual unidimensional scales (as are IRT/Rasch models). In contrast, health outcomes measures may be seeking to estimate the effects of many dimensions, with a need for a measure of the relative and combined effect of such dimensions.
- The CTT approach does not provide interval measures. Chapter 8 describes how Rasch/IRT models deal with the same issues.

Thurstone's methods

Thurstone's Method of Equal-appearing Intervals:

- The Method of Equal-appearing Intervals is a direct model where items are rated directly by the subject (and most commonly by a group of subjects), the rating or average forming the scale value of the item. This method was employed in the formation of the Sickness Impact Profile or SIP.

Thurstone's Law of Comparative Judgment and the Method of Paired Comparisons:

- Thurstone's Law of Comparative Judgement produced a probabilistic indirect method for developing interval scales, which led directly to modern indirect models such as the Rasch model. While greatly time consuming (with 50 items, each judge would need to make 1225 judgments) and relatively complex, the procedure produces an interval scale.

Guttman's 'deterministic' model

The potential advantages of the item response options that form Guttman scales over Likert scales are:

- Guttman scales employ multiple options that together clearly define the area being assessed and so reduce ambiguity (and hence reduce error).
- the individual item-options themselves can be extensively described and operationalized, and hence further reduce misunderstanding and error.
- every item-option can have a different score; hence equal differences between item response options are not assumed.

The Guttman scale is a link to modern test theory where the deterministic step function has been replaced with a more realistic probabilistic ogive.

KEY POINTS

- CTT defines the strength of the attribute (or ability) in terms of the observed score, in contrast to modern test theory, which estimates the strength of the attribute in terms of the underlying, latent trait.
- Classical tests assume that an observed test or item score can be decomposed into a 'true' score representing the value of the attribute, and an 'error' score. Because the error is by definition random, the more items that are averaged, the more the average approaches the amount of the attribute, as the summed errors will approach zero.
- In CTT, test reliability indicates the proportion of test variability that is due to error variance. Note, however, that a test is not reliable or unreliable: reliability is a property of the scores on a test for a particular group of subjects; reliability coefficients apply only to the group upon which the test was developed.
- There can be a tradeoff between test reliability and test validity. Overly homogeneous tests may be more reliable but may also provide poor estimates of a heterogenous concept (such as HQoL).
- CTT (and Modern Test Theory) is focused on the formation of individual unidimensional scales. Health outcomes measures

may be seeking to assess the effects of many dimensions, and may require sub-tests that estimate the individual dimensions plus an estimate of the combined effect of all the dimensions.

- Classical tests are relatively straightforward to create, but according to proponents of Modern Test Theory, they do not provide interval measures (see Ch. 8). Thurston's Law of Comparative Judgement and Guttman scales have links to Modern Test Theory.

Steps in developing a classical test

AIMS OF CHAPTER

- To provide a practically orientated account of steps in developing a classical test

- To provide practical examples for a number of the steps

- To review key issues in traditional test development

FINALIZE ISSUES CONCERNING THE NATURE OF THE TEST

The issues to be resolved are the purpose and construct of the test, and the criteria the test needs to meet (see Ch. 3). These should include the following:

Who is to provide the information and ratings (e.g. of health states) that may be needed in test development?

As described in Chapter 1, tests vary in the extent that they rely on information or assessments from patients versus others. For measures of health-related quality of life (QoL), patient report is the primary source of data (see Ch. 5), although adaptation (Ch. 2) may require that the judgements of others also be included.

Is the test to be unidimensional or multidimensional?

There is considerable merit in assessing dimensions individually, as it aids interpretation of the results. Which dimensions should be assessed cannot be concluded until after an extensive process of consulting literature, patients, healthcare personnel, and others. Heterogeneous elements are desirable. Feinstein (1999) noted that the five component variables selected for the Apgar scale were chosen because they were heterogeneous elements, each making a different contribution to the final sum.

Inclusion of a global question

Inclusion of a global question to be answered by the patient, or whoever is completing the questionnaire, is highly recommended. It allows unconsidered but important variables to express themselves and provides a means of checking whether the items were interpreted as intended (see Ch. 5 under 'Patient Global Self-ratings').

The cognitive demands of the test

Excessive cognitive demand of the task may lead to confused responses. The more complex the execution of the test, the more likely the test will be reflecting patients' cognitive abilities and not their health state. Hanita (2000), for example, suggests that utility advocates in particular need to develop measures that are less taxing of patients. See Chapter 5 under 'Avoid Overly Complex Tasks', and Chapter 4 under 'Validity Evidence Related to the Test Tasks'.

How generic/specific is the test?

There is merit in developing instruments that are hybrids (and this may commonly be the case, see Shumaker et al 1997).

Including a global question will allow an illness-specific instrument to have some of the virtues of generic instruments.

The role of a criterion such as patient self-assessed health-related quality of life

Most HQoL tests should be criterion-orientated. There is a criterion by definition, namely 'the patients' assessment of their own health'. The process of developing an instrument allows this to be built into the test. Patient self-assessment may be better viewed as a proxy-criterion, not a gold standard (e.g. given the complex nature of adaptation). Other tests might pursue a criterion of expert judgement, or an objective variable observable in the future (e.g. likelihood of readmission to hospital).

DETERMINE THE CONTENT OF THE TEST

The process of developing appropriate content includes:

- Review of research, including examination of literature regarding the conditions targeted and similar instruments.
- Consultation with healthcare workers with first-hand professional experience of the effects of the illness.
- Discussion with patients, ideally individually, although group meetings can also be beneficial.
- For patients whose illness makes interview difficult, direct observation and examination of clinical records.

Open ended questions posed to patients generate a great deal of important information, often more than is found through the literature or discussion with healthcare personnel. Statements made in unstructured interviews also can be turned readily into items, as they have the advantage of being expressed in the everyday language of the respondents themselves (as opposed to being contrived by the researcher; see Moser & Kalton 1979). Haig et al (1989) asked subjects to describe in narrative form their most recent and most severe illness, and to write about the types of discomfort or unpleasant sensations they experienced during the course of a day.

Content should be comprehensive. Shumaker et al (1997) suggested that a HQoL measure needs to be able to capture both the complex natural history of the disease, the effects associated with the disease's progression, and its treatment both positive and negative. There might also be augmentation with carefully developed symptom checklists.

Sensitive issues may need to be explored. Feinstein (1999) observed that sexual activity was not included among items used to rate functional status before receiving a hip replacement, and while sex may not be pertinent for some elderly patients, it may for others be the standard for assessing the operation's success.

Candidate test materials and their contained dimensions may be checked with patients to ensure they are meaningful and relevant, and to determine which items/materials seem most relevant (Donovan et al 1989).

DETERMINE THE WORDING OF EACH ITEM

Both validity and reliability depend ultimately on the characteristics of individual items. High reliability and validity can be built into the test through item qualitative and quantitative analysis, followed by the selection, substitution and revision of items.

Drafting items

Items need to be prepared carefully and revised extensively in terms of their content and form. Ideally, items will be expressed in natural language, i.e. the language of the patients.

In drafting items, it is important to minimize ambiguity. This is reduced by operationalizing items, i.e. using concrete examples instead of terms such as 'severely' and 'moderately'. Thus 'seriously disruptive' becomes 'disrupts work for at least 60 minutes per day'.

It is important to consider the way items are framed (see Ch. 5 under 'No Scaling Is Direct: There Are Effects of Instruction: Stimuli and Response', and 'Be Aware of Framing Effects').

Traditionally, there have been relatively few texts available to advise on item writing (and new challenges have emerged with the uptake of Item Response Theory (IRT)) (Cella & Chang 2000). However, Frary (1996a) provides useful advice, including the following:

1. Define precisely the information desired and endeavour to write as few questions as possible to obtain it.
2. Obtain feedback on the initial list of questions, e.g. from a small but representative sample of potential responders, with

a field trial of a tentative form of the questionnaire also desirable.

3. Locate personal or confidential questions at the end of the questionnaire, as early unsettling questions may cause respondents to not continue.
4. Order response categories so that a progression between a lower level of response and a higher is listed in left-to-right order, i.e. (1) Never, (2) Seldom, (3) Occasionally, (4) Frequently.
5. Consider combining categories, e.g. combining 'seldom' with 'never' if responders would be very unlikely to mark 'never' and 'seldom' would connote almost equal activity.
6. Ask responders to rate both positive and negative stimuli, otherwise the respondent may be encouraged to uniformly agree or disagree to all of the responses.
7. Choose appropriate response category language and logic – where views are likely to be clear then: (1) Agree, (2) Disagree may be suitable, but when opinions may not be strong use: (1) Agree, (2) Tend to agree, (3) Tend to disagree, (4) Disagree.

For further advice on questionnaire design, see Frary (1996b), Hinkle et al (1985), and Haladyna & Downing (1988a, b). Mullin et al (2000) present guidelines for the formatting of HQoL questionnaires.

Select the response scales for each item

There are many ways of presenting items. Common ways are via Guttman and Likert formats, as well as dichotomous items (e.g. yes/no) and visual analogue scales (VAS).

There is no obvious reason why different types of item-response scales cannot be combined in a test. In fact there are arguments in favour of heterogeneity of methods. For example, items measuring different constructs but with the same scale response formats could lead to spurious correlations (due to common methods variance), while mixing formats such as using both VAS scales and Likert scales could encourage respondents to think more carefully about what is being asked of them (Gardner et al 1998). Items can also be keyed in both directions and cover multiple situations (Nunnally & Bernstein 1994). Equal numbers of 'yes' and 'no' answers may reduce acquiescence bias or agreement with the statement (although, see Smith 1996).

Pretest items for clarity and comprehensibility

Following initial development, items need to be tested and refined. Pre-testing items entails presenting them to the type of subjects the test is designed for, and testing that they are comprehensible, unambiguous, and ask only a single question.

It is essential to confirm that subjects understand the items the way they are intended. This 'cognitive de-briefing' may entail asking subjects to think aloud as they complete the draft questionnaire. It is almost guaranteed that items will need to be deleted, added, or re-written.

This can be an arduous process, that needs to be repeated a number of times.

Where applicable, scale items (e.g. for Guttman scale items)

Depending upon the types of items being developed, the scaling of individual item responses may be needed. This is generally necessary when developing Guttman scales, but can be applied to any response scale (e.g. Likert) where verbal labels are used.

For example, in one study, the response scale 'never', 'not usually', 'sometimes', 'usually', 'always' was used to assess availability of domiciliary support services. In analyzing the data, concerns were expressed that these responses might not be equally separated on the underlying continuum. To investigate, the staff who had completed the questionnaire were asked to place these same labels on a scale of 0–100. The average values given were 0, 17, 36, 73, 100. In other words, the adjacent labels 'not usually' and 'sometimes' were judged to be relatively close, compared to the adjacent labels 'sometimes' and 'usually' (Rembicki, personal communication).

As pointed out by Spector (1976), the selection of response categories is often arbitrary with the equal interval properties of the consequent response continuum assumed inappropriately.

It is suggested that scale values be routinely checked, and the determined values used or the response labels changed to ones indicating more equal spacing. The easiest way to scale items is via some form of category rating scale (Ch. 5), such as a VAS or a variant of Thurstone's Method of Equal-appearing Intervals (Ch. 6).

As noted earlier, the selection of the most appropriate scaling task can be a controversial issue. Economists and psychologists have traditionally differed in their preferred approaches to scaling health states (Kaplan et al 1993). Those with a background in psychology and education are more likely to embrace rating scales, while health economists have traditionally favoured techniques that include uncertainty (such as the Standard Gamble, although this has now declined in popularity, see Richardson 1997). There is increasing recognition among health economists that psychometric methods may have advantages. See Chapter 11 under 'Measuring Utilities'.

The use of expert judges

The use of expert judges to gather ratings and scale items raises the question of how many judges, and how to respond when they disagree. These issues do not seem to have been satisfactorily resolved.

Edwards & Fasolo (2001) observed that some information is obtainable only by expert judgement, and the most lively disagreements are what to do when experts differ. In the context of gathering expert probability estimates they suggested the options were:

1. pick one expert
2. average functions or parameters across experts
3. discuss and then re-elicit, or
4. elicit a single agreed-on estimate from the experts working together face-to-face.

They noted neither experimentation nor extensive experience (e.g. in gathering daily weather forecasts) had provided unambiguous guidance about what to do when experts disagree.

In the practical experience of the author, the consensus option (4.) above is less satisfactory than a process of identifying and excluding the most deviant judges, and then averaging responses. This process was followed in the revision and final development of the Work Ability Tables (O'Connor et al 1996). See Box 7.1.

CONDUCT QUANTITATIVE ITEM ANALYSIS

Items can be analyzed quantitatively, in terms of their statistical properties, to increase the test's validity and reliability. Other things being equal, a test with more items is more valid and reliable

---

Box 7.1   Rewording and rescaling items: The Work Ability Tables (WATs)

Items forming a health measurement scale need to be clear and unambiguous, and their values need to reflect their importance. An example is the items making up the Work Ability Tables (WATs). The first version of the WATs sub-scales had been developed by Shane Thomas and Maree Dyson of La Trobe University. Items had been selected so as to be relevant to generic domains of work ability, and as far as possible relevant to all forms of work.

However, validation studies suggested the instrument might fail to accurately measure ability to work, and further development and evaluation of the tables was conducted (O'Connor et al 1996). The first step was to ensure that each item was precise and unambiguous, the aim being to minimize sources of error variance that might diminish reliability and validity.

The types of changes introduced included:

(a) *operationalizing definitions*, e.g. 'some reduction in dexterity' was given the example of 'difficulty smoothly placing key in lock'.

(b) *explicitly quantifying phrases* by removing terms such as 'severely' and 'moderately', thus 'seriously disruptive' became 'disrupts work for at least 60 minutes per day'.

(c) *clarifying and emphasizing the domain*, e.g. stressing that communication difficulties refers to sensory impairment, but not to cognitive impairment or language knowledge.

The values given to the WAT descriptors had previously been agreed in a committee situation, but never subjected to formal scaling. For the WATs to be valid, the scores needed as far as possible to have interval properties.

To check the interval properties of the descriptors, i.e. that score values reflected a descriptor's position on the linear scale of 'no reduction in ability to work' to 'totally unable to work', each of the new modified descriptors was presented to 30 medical officers for rating. The items were presented in two different orders, and the ratings made using a visual rating scale of 0 to 100, where 0 signified no disability for work, and 100 represented total disability for work. The results of the rating exercise are provided in Figure 7.1.

It can be seen that the scaling exercise led to quite marked departures from the initial, informal scaling. For example, of 8 items which had been given an equal score of '5' in informal scaling, the same items produced a 2:1 range of values when scaled formally, ranging from '20' to '40'.

---

than a short test (the effect of shortening a test on reliability was discussed earlier, and the Spearman-Brown formula can be applied to estimate this effect).

When a test is shortened by eliminating the least satisfactory items, it can be both more valid and reliable, and shorter than the original. This applies as long as all the items are targeting the same unidimensional construct. If not, multiple sub-scales will be needed to develop overall test validity.

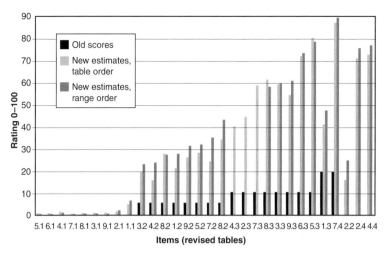

Figure 7.1   Comparison of old and new scores for 'ability to work'.

Item difficulty

When developing a sum-scale (see Ch. 6), after pre-testing for readability and absence of ambiguity, the set of items may be given to a large group of subjects to test for other attributes including endorsement frequency (Streiner & Norman 1996 suggest 50 subjects as a minimum). The frequency of endorsement is the proportion of people who select each response alternative for an item. For dichotomous items this is the proportion of 'yes' or 'no', and in a multiple-choice item, it is the proportion choosing alternative A, alternative B, etc.

Item alternatives receiving very high or low endorsement rates are then generally eliminated (certainly 100% or 0%). With such items, little is learnt by knowing how a person responded, i.e. such questions do not improve a scale's properties, they only make the test longer.

Streiner & Norman suggest that only items with endorsement rates between 0.20 and 0.80 be used, while Anastasi (1990) recommends the selection of items with a moderate spread of difficulty, and with an average difficulty level overall of 0.50 (i.e. an average endorsement of 50%).

Note there can be scales made of items that deliberately have a high expected endorsement frequency, e.g. those aimed at determining the subject's ability or willingness to answer honestly.

Item discrimination

As described in Chapter 6, item discrimination is the capacity of an item to discriminate between high and low ability testees in the behaviour or attribute that the test is designed to measure. This can be signaled in two ways: by the item correlating highly with the total test score, and by the item correlating highly with an external criterion.

Item correlation with the total test score

A discriminating item is more likely to be endorsed by a person who has a high total score than by someone with a low total score, i.e. the item discriminates between those who score high and hence are supposed to have more of the trait, and those who score low. Hence item discrimination can be indicated by the degree to which the score on the item correlates with the total test score.

Item correlation with a criterion

When the test as a whole is evaluated by means of *criterion-related validation,* items may be evaluated and selected on the basis of their relationship to the same external criterion. Anastasi (1990) describes how this procedure has a particular role in the development of attitude tests, which HQoL measures largely correspond to. In contrast to choosing items on the basis of correlation with total test score, which tends to maximize the internal consistency or homogeneity of the test, doing so based on correlation with an external criterion maximizes the validity of the test against the external criterion.

Item-total correlation and criterion correlation may lead to opposite results

Under certain conditions, the two approaches may lead to opposite results. That is, the items chosen on the basis of external validity may be the very ones rejected on the basis of internal consistency (Anastasi 1990). The reason for this is that selecting items that have high correlations with total test score means items with the highest average inter-correlations will be retained. This method of selecting items *will increase test validity only when the original pool of items measures a single trait and when this trait is represented by the criterion.* However, some pools of items measure a combination of attributes that is required by a complex criterion. Purifying the test in this case using item-total correlation may reduce its criterion coverage, and lower validity.

This is just the situation that is likely to occur in HQoL measurement, if an attempt is made to place items assessing mobility, depression, sociability, etc. in a single scale.

In fact, external validation and internal consistency are both desirable objectives of test construction, and the relative emphasis to be placed on each varies with the nature and purpose of the test (Nunnally & Bernstein 1994 [pp. 320–322] take a less accepting view).

Resolving the dilemma: homogeneity within sub-tests, and heterogeneity between sub-tests

A satisfactory compromise is to sort the relatively homogeneous items into separate tests or sub-tests, each of which covers a different aspect of the external criterion. Then breadth of coverage can be achieved through a variety of tests, each yielding a relatively unambiguous score, rather than through heterogeneity of items within a single test. Internal consistency would be attained within each sub-test or item group, and validity of the overall test (i.e. battery of sub-scales) would be developed through an appropriate sub-scale combination rule (Anastasi 1990).

Techniques used to assess item difficulty and item discrimination: coefficient alpha and factor analysis

The interactive use of statistical programmes that compute item-total correlations and coefficient alpha can play a useful role in identifying items with unsuitable item difficulty and item discrimination properties. However, for the reasons already discussed, basing item selection solely on item-total correlations can lead to significant problems for a test that needs heterogeneous items for adequate assessment (such as HQoL).

Factor analysis can play a role in determining whether a set of items is actually measuring a number of different concepts (e.g. see Cohen & Swerdlick 1999). Items loading on different factors may need to be separated into sub-tests and tests of item difficulty applied (see Anastasi 1990, Anastasi & Urbina 1997).

DEVELOPING A METHOD FOR COMBINING SUB-TEST SCORES

If an instrument assesses multiple HQoL domains via multiple sub-scales, a method of combining sub-scale score will be needed if there is to be an index overall. Various tools are available to assist with this, such as multiple regression or logistic regression (see Ch. 4 under 'The Role of Multiple Regression in HQoL Measurement').

As the most important domains are likely to vary depending upon the illness state being assessed, a scoring method that selectively weights certain domains may be best for measuring the global effects of a particular illness (note that the presence or absence of a domain is the most profound form of weighting).

However, the rule may not be simple. As discussed in Chapter 2 under 'The Global Evaluation of an Experienced State Is Not the Sum of Its Parts', the reported well-being/HQoL of an experienced state tends not to be predicted by a simple amalgamation of its parts. Instead, key elements are abstracted from the experience, such as the most intense part of the experience and the nature of the end of the experience (Redelmeier & Kahneman 1996). Further evidence suggested a related principle may apply when multiple qualitatively different sources of stress are acting. Thus Bergner et al (1976a) found that judges estimating overall patient dysfunction appeared to attend to both the range of dysfunction and the most severe dysfunctions. Similarly, O'Connor et al (1996, see below) found that the best predictor of global work-related disability, as rated by medical officers, was the score of the highest-rated disability of the patient.

In other words, there is evidence of a tendency to focus on salient features, not to simply sum all sources. A discount scoring system may be the most predictive, e.g. where overall HQoL is governed by the most disabling domain, not a simple sum of all domains.

The Work Ability Tables (WATs)

The Work Ability Tables (WATs) (O'Connor et al 1996) were developed to help assess eligibility for pensions. The WATs scoring

Table 7.1   Correlations between scoring measure and % global estimates of 'inability to carry out usual work'

Measure	Global estimate
Maximum score among sub-tables	0.61
Total of all sub-tables	0.52
No. sub-table scores > 0	0.47

system was developed by determining which method of combining nine sub-scale scores best predicted 'Global Inability to Work' estimated by medical officers after examining the patient.

A number of score types were investigated, some of which are presented in Table 7.1.

It is apparent that the measure correlating most highly with the global estimate was the maximum score among sub-tables. The result of subsequent analyses was that the most effective and efficient combination could be approximated by: Work-ability = Max. value + 10 × (Number of values > 0) − 0.1 × (Max. value × No. > 0). This indicates that the judgement of medical officers concerning 'able/unable' to work may be best represented by a rule that considers the maximum degree of disability experienced in any one area, and the degree of spread of disability across different disability areas.

Note that to use a scoring system based on selecting the highest scoring items, it is necessary that all items in all domains are scaled against one clearly defined standard.

TRAINING IN THE TEST

Tests that require to be administered can require training of the administrators. Tests that require significant training for administration should be avoided if possible, as there is no guarantee that such training will always be available or completed. Training is also likely to be of varying effectiveness (cf. Lumley & McNamara 1995).

DEVELOPING INTERPRETABILITY

The implications of differences in test score need to be judged carefully, raising the general matter of how to interpret the size of a difference. With health status tests, the term 'interpretability' is commonly used, i.e. the degree to which one can assign qualitative meaning to an instrument's quantitative scores. This is an issue in both research and clinical settings (although recently more prominent in clinical ones).

General population norms

Scores on psychological tests are often interpreted by reference to norms that represent the test performance relevant to a standardization sample. The norms are empirically established by determining what the individuals in a representative group actually do on the test. Any individual's raw score can then be referred to the distribution of scores obtained by the standardization sample, to discover where he or she falls in that distribution (see Anastasi 1990). Such an approach is applicable to tests that aim to assess individuals vis a vis a stable general population, but is less suitable with illness-specific tests and a clinical population.

Clinical populations

Kazis et al (1989) suggested that differences in mean scores (from baseline to test) should be related to the standard deviation of the scores at the baseline (see also Guyatt et al 2002). Deyo & Patrick (1989) suggested that such an index could be used to calculate a 'responsiveness coefficient', which would indicate the smallest clinically important score change for an instrument.

In general, translating a quantitative score to a qualitative category that has clinical or commonly understood meaning can be aided by:

- information on the relationship of scores to clinically recognized conditions or need for specific treatments
- comparative data on the distribution of scores derived from a variety of defined population groups, including a representative sample of the general population
- relating changes in scores to commonly recognized life events (such as the impact of losing a job) or relevant healthcare events such as need for institutional care.

These issues are discussed further in Chapter 11 under 'Interpreting Quality of Life Scores for Individual Patients'.

SUMMARY

Finalize issues concerning the nature of the test

- Who is to provide the information and ratings that may be needed in test development?
- Is the test to be unidimensional or multidimensional?
- Will a global question be included?
- The cognitive demands of the test.
- How generic/specific is the test to be?
- The role of a criterion such as patient self-assessed HQoL.

Determine the content of the test

- Review of research.
- Consultation with healthcare, examination of clinical records.
- Discussion with patients.
- Observation for patients for whom interview is difficult (e.g. dementia).

Determine the wording of each item

Draft items:

- Express items in the language of the patients.
- Operationalize items to minimize ambiguity.

Select the item/response scale type:

- Dichotomous, Guttman, Likert, VAS.
- Be aware of possible response biases (minimized by different item types?).
- Heterogenity is desirable.

Pre-test items for clarity and comprehensibility:

- Confirm that subjects understand the items in the way that they were intended.
- Delete, add, re-write, repeat pre-testing.

Where applicable, scale items, as for Guttman scales:

- The easiest way to scale items is via a VAS, or Thurstone's Method of Equal-appearing Intervals.
- Consider use of expert judges.

Examination of quantitative item analysis

Item difficulty – eliminate item alternatives that everyone or no-one selects.

Item discrimination ('the capacity of an item to discriminate between high and low ability testees') can be assessed by:

- Item correlation with the total test score: Item discrimination can be indicated by the degree to which the score on the item correlates with the total test score.
- Item correlation with a criterion: Items may also be selected on the basis of their relationship to an external criterion.

Item-total correlation and criterion correlation may lead to opposite results when the items are multidimensional.

- Resolve the dilemma by homogeneity within sub-tests and heterogeneity between sub-tests.
- The development of unidimensional scales may be assisted by coefficient alpha and factor analysis.

Develop a method for combining sub-test scores

Instruments that assess multiple HQoL domains via multiple sub-scales will need a rule to estimate overall HQoL. Multiple regression or logistic regression can help. The rule may not be simple, as:

- Reported well-being of an experienced state tends not to be a simple amalgamation of its parts (Redelmeier & Kahneman 1996, Bergner et al 1976a, O'Connor et al 1996).
- Overall HQoL may be governed by the most distressing domain, not a simple sum of all.

Training in the test

Tests that require significant training for administration should be avoided. There is no guarantee that training will always be available, completed, or have lasting effect.

Develop interpretability

Population norms can be used when assessing individuals vis a vis a general population, but are less suitable for a clinical population.

Translating a quantitative score to a commonly understood meaning can be aided by:

- information on the relationship of scores to clinically recognized conditions or need for specific treatments
- comparative data on the distribution of scores derived from a variety of defined population groups
- relating changes in scores to commonly recognized life events (such as the impact of losing a job) or relevant healthcare events such as need for institutional care.

FURTHER POINTS

- Developing a classical test is not difficult, but developing a good classical test is; moreover, the test will have faults. It is important that the test developer does not rest on her/his laurels, but is among the first to point out shortcomings and ways to improve.
- The success of the test should not be judged by whether it is used by others in the health industry – when the test meets a need, health professionals will be only too ready to adopt it – but whether it accurately predicts or estimates what it is intended to. This means a further programme of testing and evaluation, comparing its output to the best direct measures of the attribute available, for each population it is intended to be used with.

QUOTABLE QUOTE

No amount of statistical manipulation after the fact can compensate for poorly chosen questions; those that are badly worded, ambiguous, irrelevant, or – even worse – not present.

(Streiner & Norman 1996, p. 15)

Modern test theory

AIMS OF CHAPTER

- To outline the arguments regarding the importance of interval
  properties for psychological variables, and why classical
  approaches are claimed to be deficient

- Introduce Item Response Theory (IRT) and the Rasch model,
  and contrast them with classical approaches

- Explain the merits of tests based on the Rasch model

- Provide an overview of the elements entailed in forming a Rasch-based test

- Further explore the issue of developing tests based on multiple dimensions

Modern Test Theory, represented by Item Response Theory (IRT) and the Rasch model, holds that classical tests fail to adequately quantify the attributes they seek to measure, i.e. they lack interval properties. Before introducing Modern Test Theory, the debate on why interval properties are necessary and how they may be achieved is outlined.

SHOULD ESTIMATES OF PSYCHOLOGICAL ATTRIBUTES HAVE INTERVAL MEASUREMENT PROPERTIES?

The statistical view: measures of constructs do not need interval properties

Until recently, the common de facto view was that measures of human attributes do not need to have interval properties (here termed the 'statistical' view, versus the 'representational' view – after Gaito, see Nunnally & Bernstein 1994). Indeed, it has been argued that no psychological scale may be interval, in the sense that equal quantities at different parts of the scale are meaningfully equivalent ('intelligence', say, as opposed to 'length'). The primary question has instead been seen to be 'what do we want to measure', and 'how do we measure it so that responses can legitimately aid decision-making'.

In this view, a response scale need not possess interval properties to be useful in health status measurement, and that while most if not all psychological variables are in fact ordinal, they may *quite justifiably* be treated as if they were interval or ratio variables for statistical purposes.

For example, Ferguson (1966) noted that in the analysis of statistical data in psychology and education, it is common for the information to be superimposed on the data, e.g. to assume that a set of ordinal numbers is interval and proceed to apply arithmetic operations to these numbers. Ferguson suggested that scores on intelligence tests, attitude tests and personality tests are all in effect ordinal variables, because no aspect of the operation of measuring intelligence, say, permits the making of meaningful statements about the equality of intervals. Thus it cannot be said that the differences in intelligence between a person with an IQ of 80 and one with an IQ of 90 is in any sense equal to the difference in intelligence between a person with an IQ of 110 and one with 120. Much the same argument could be applied to a health-related quality of life (HQoL) scale.

Although a purist might conclude that statistical techniques that require interval properties should not be applied to such data, Ferguson disagreed, maintaining that practical necessity can dictate a procedure, although it should be understood what assumptions are being made.

A second and related argument, is that most parametric statistical tests do not require data to be measured on an interval scale, but rather that tests require assumptions about the distribution of the data: parametric statistics can be used as long as the data meets these distribution assumptions. For example, Anderson (1976) proposed that the concern with interval or linear scales is unnecessary in many applications, as the power of a statistical test has no necessary relation to the nature of the response scale.

Some have responded to this view by testing whether the distribution is normal, and then correcting non-normal data using transformations (cf. Hall et al 1989).

Others have been even more pragmatic. Crocker & Algina (1986) concluded that psychology test data should be treated as interval scale data as long as it can be demonstrated empirically that usefulness of the scores for prediction or description is enhanced by this treatment. Stevens who popularized the ordinal/interval debate was quoted as sanctioning the use of parametric statistics on the pragmatic grounds that it can lead to fruitful results.

Shavelson (1988) in a text on statistical reasoning for behavioural science, illustrated the hands-off approach of most to this issue, in arguing that the problem was not of matching statistical methods as interpreting the results, quoting Hays in that 'the experimenting psychologist [sociologist, educational researcher] must face the problem of the interpretation of statistical results within psychology and on extra-mathematical grounds' (Hays 1973, p. 88).

The 'representational' view: measures of constructs can and should have interval properties

An alternative school has argued that measures of psychological constructs must possess interval properties if the study of human behaviour is to become a science. Advocates of this 'representational' view argue that the 'statistical' view has led to the acceptance of poor quality tests, and the acceptance of standards of measurement that physics (say) would consider totally unacceptable.

Michell (1997) argued this view vigorously, noting that in 1940, the non-psychologist members of a committee established by the British Association for the Advancement of Science agreed that psychophysical methods did not constitute scientific measurement, the primary reason given by the Association being that the additivity of psychological attributes had not been displayed and so there was no evidence to support the hypothesis that psychophysical methods measured anything.

Michell maintained that this was a legitimate criticism and one that still applied, that the definition of measurement endorsed in practice by quantitative psychologists (those who theorize about or attempt to measure psychological quantities) was as formulated by Stevens (1946), namely 'measurement is the assignment of numerals to objects or events according to rule'. In other words, the need for measures to have interval properties, i.e. to be additive, was being ignored. (For further discussion and some opposing arguments, refer to the *British Journal of Psychology*, vol 38, issue 3, August 1997.)

Michell further maintained that this position had been unnecessary ever since the development of the *theory of conjoint measurement* (Luce & Tukey 1964). Conjoint measurement is concerned with the way an additive variable can be constructed via a monotonic transformation of an ordinal measure: when certain axioms hold, and the ordering of a dependent variable varies with the joint effect of two or more independent variables, the transformed dependent variable and the concomitantly constructed independent variables are simultaneously (hence 'conjoint') considered to be represented on an interval scale with a common unit. In essence, an additive representation is achieved without the existence of an empirical concatenation operation (Perline et al 1979). ' … when no natural concatenation operation exists, one should try to discover a way to measure factors and responses such that the 'effects' of different factors are additive ... ' (Luce & Tukey 1964, p. 4).

The result of the theory of conjoint measurement was that measurement, as when physical quantities such as height and weight are combined, was shown to be a theoretical property, one that could be realized in the behavioural and biological sciences to produce interval and ratio scales (Wright 1997b, Luce & Tukey 1964). In other words, psychological and behavioural measures (such as measures of HQoL) could possess interval properties if they met the requirements of conjoint additivity.

Finally, it has been argued that conjoint additivity is practically expressed in the Rasch psychometric model, i.e. the Rasch model provides an additive framework and hence can produce measures that achieve interval properties. 'The Rasch model is an example of conjoint measurement that has an underlying stochastic [i.e. probabilistic] structure ... which can be applied to empirical data and tested for goodness-of-fit using the general procedures of statistical inference' (Perline et al 1979, p. 238; see also Wright 1997a,b, 1999, Embretson 1996).

At the coal face: ignoring interval properties leads to perceptibly poor items

Vague, indeterminate, or unequal response categories seem often to be part of scales intended to measure health-related behaviour.

Wright (1997a) referred to the measurement of outcomes in rehabilitation, where patients may be assessed on tasks of daily living by use of ratings such as 1) Maximally dependent, 2) Moderate assistance, and 3) Minimal assistance. Wright points out that while a rating of 2 would seem more than a rating of 1, it is not clear by how much. Yet such ratings are analyzed as if they differ by 1 unit each.

Feinstein (1999) in discussing the Apgar scale noted that previously, a baby's condition tended to be described with ratings such as excellent, good, fair or poor, or with phrases such as mild, moderate or severe. He observed that the interpretation of such ratings was heavily influenced by individual judgment, and that such ratings were often unreliable and idiosyncratic.

The difficulty in accepting items at their stated value applies also to dichotomous items (e.g. those requiring 'yes' or 'no'). Hence a 'carer sleeplessness' scale might include 'carer has less than eight hours sleep', 'carer verbally reassures patient several times each night', 'carer toilets patient two to three times every night'. While some suggest more of a problem than others, on a sum scale, each would be scored '0' or '1' and then totalled.

Similarly, within a test, all Likert scale items and response categories (e.g. 'Strongly agree', 'Agree', 'Neither agree nor disagree', 'Disagree', 'Strongly disagree') are treated as if on the same interval scale, differing by one unit. However, such items can bias participants' responses toward the centre points of the scale (Harrison & McLaughlin 1993), while equivalent Likert responses in a test (e.g. 'Strongly agree' on one item and 'Strongly agree' on another) can correspond to different levels of the same attribute (e.g. see Bond & Fox 2001).

The result of the preceding combination of theoretical and in-practice concerns has been a gradual but ongoing move toward test models that pursue measures with interval properties (a good deal of work by researchers such as Thurstone in the first half of the 20th century presaged this shift, as described in Ch. 6). The following outlines the nature of these models – the latent trait models.

LATENT TRAIT MODELS: ITEM RESPONSE THEORY AND THE RASCH MODEL

As described earlier, classical tests treat all items as equivalent, and estimate the level of the attribute by summing all positive responses (i.e. those indicating possession of the attribute).

In contrast, tests based on latent trait theory maintain that positively scoring a given item requires a unique minimum level of the attribute, and as a result, modelling and evaluating the *pattern* of responses is needed to identify the person's level of the attribute (not simply totalling them).

Item Response Theory (IRT) Models and the Rasch model are members of this group, as is the Guttman scale (although the scale is a deterministic not a probabilistic version).

In one sense, the Rasch model is merely the simplest (one-parameter logistic [1PL]) of the models that make up IRT. In another sense, it represents a unique philosophy of test construction, as its fiercest advocates hold that alone among the IRT family of models, it produces tests that meet the requirements of scientific measurement (see 'The Difference between Rasch and IRT' later in this chapter).

Item characteristic curves, difficulty and discrimination

As described by Nunnally & Bernstein (1994), IRT and the Rasch model can be represented by the notion of the item-characteristic curve (ICC), which relates the probability of a 'correct' response to an item (i.e. a response indicating more of the trait) to the strength of an underlying trait.

In essence, the more of the attribute that a person possesses, the more likely it is that an item that signals possession of the attribute will be confirmed. However, the model is probabilistic: it is more likely but not certain. The likelihood of the item being affirmed is indicated by the difficulty and discrimination of the item, as well as the ability (strength of attribute) of the person. In IRT/Rasch models the difficulty and discrimination of an item are represented as basic properties of an ICC trace line.

The ICC may be a cumulative normal distribution, but is typically assumed to be a logistic ogive (see Fig. 8.1), and always for the Rasch model.

To appreciate the nature of latent trait theory it is necessary to understand how the item parameters of *difficulty* and *discrimination* are viewed in these models.

In latent trait terms, difficulty refers to how much of the attribute a person must have if they are to successfully complete the item (and so suggest they possess at least that corresponding level of the attribute). For example, in a test of anxiety, agreement with the item would tend to suggest some minimum level of anxiety. In IRT, difficulty is defined as the amount of the attribute necessary to have a 0.5 probability of passing the item. In Figure 8.1, Item 'b' has the same difficulty as the Reference item, but less difficulty than Item 'a'.

The 'discrimination' of an item describes the extent to which the probability of passing the item correlates with the strength of the attribute. An item with a perfectly flat trace line would not discriminate, and hence cannot signal the presence of the attribute and has no value in the test. In Figure 8.1, Item 'b' has the greatest discrimination (the steepest ascending trace), while the Reference item and Item 'a' have equal (and lesser) discrimination.

Generally, it is assumed that the probability of passing the item will increase with the strength of the attribute (a monotonic function). In terms of the ICC, making an item more discriminating increases its slope.

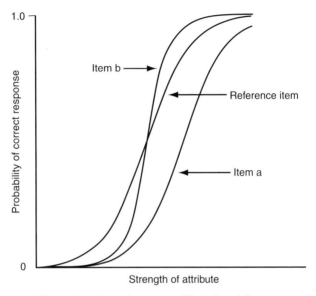

Figure 8.1 Effects of making an item more difficult (item 'a') or more discriminating (item 'b') relative to a reference item (adapted with permission from Nunnally J C, Bernstein I H 1994 Psychometric theory, 3rd edn, © McGraw-Hill Companies, Inc.).

In general, IRT and the Rasch model use information from item trace lines that relate strength of attribute to the probability of a response. The location (threshold) of the trace line defines the difficulty of the item, and the slope defines the item's ability to discriminate.

In terms of analyzing a test, a key requirement is to estimate the parameters of the items. Once the parameters of the trace lines of all items in the test have been estimated, the relationship between the level of the attribute held by a person completing the test and the probability of a given item response pattern (which items were correct if dichotomous, or which had higher scores if Likert scales) is known, and hence the attribute strength for any person completing the test can be estimated.

The latent trait family: 1PL Item Response Theory and Rasch 2PL IRT, 3PL IRT

1. The simplest one-parameter logistic (1PL) model IRT and the Rasch model assume that items vary only with respect to their

difficulty, i.e. all have the same discrimination, and guessing is not taken into account. Note that the Guttman scale is a special case of this model where the items are both of equal discrimination and *perfectly* discriminating, i.e. the slope of the trace line is vertical. For this model, the classical measure of performance (number of correct responses) is sufficient to estimate the value of the trait.

2. The next simplest IRT model is the two-parameter model (2PL), where items may vary in both discrimination and difficulty. The overall effect of guessing is still treated as insignificant.

3. In the three-parameter IRT model (3PL), items can vary with respect to discrimination, difficulty, and the probability of being guessed correctly.

Note that person ability and item difficulty are defined relative to one another, not absolutely. Both are measured on an interval scale representing the strength of attribute.

Because of limitations on the scope of this book, the following considers the Rasch/1PL IRT model only. The Rasch model is currently accepted by many to satisfy the requirements of conjoint measurement, possess interval properties, and represent the preferred guide to the development of new tests.

On the other hand, other IRT models (2PL, 3PL, etc.) are likely to be better able to characterize or describe many existing tests, as they allow and model features such as unequal discrimination and guessing. Such features exist in tests but are incompatible with interval measurement.

THE RASCH MODEL

Characteristics of the Rasch model

As described by Wright (1999), Rasch (1960, 1980) developed the Rasch model based on the notion that the probability of a person getting a correct response on an item is a function of the difference between a person's ability and an item's difficulty. This additive (interval) measurement model takes the form:

$$L = \log\left(\frac{P}{1 - P}\right) = B - D$$

L = logistic function; P = probability of a correct response and log{P/(1 − P)} = log odds of a correct response; B = person ability and D = item difficulty.

The use of the logistic function is seen to both provide an interval measure and to allow the separation of person and item parameters. This is in contrast to the normal ogive model used by Thurstone, which provides an interval measure but not separability (although numerically similar to the logistic). The logistic ICC is derived mathematically and its basic shape is determined without reference to any data. However, data are required to estimate each item's difficulty, and are examined to determine if they meet the requirements of the model (e.g. items are of similar discrimination): when there is a fit of the Rasch model, items and persons are measured on an interval scale with a common unit.

Note that perfect fit to the model requires failures on items that are easier than others that were passed. According to the Rasch (and IRT) model, if all items to the left of a point on the common logit scale (easy items) were scored correct and all to the right (harder items) were incorrect, this would not be a perfect fit. The point is that Rasch/IRT models are probabilistic; errors are expected. Indeed, if there are no errors, the scale becomes of the Guttman type, which is ordinal only. Items and persons can only be located on the underlying Rasch logit scale if there are errors to reveal their proximity (Linacre 1999).

The Rasch model is a special case of additive conjoint measurement, where conjoint additivity is a theoretical requirement for measurement (Perline et al 1979). Rasch models represent laws of quantification that define item and person independence (objective measurement), determine what is measurable, and identify which data are useful and which data are not (Wright 1999). The Rasch model is based on the specification of 'local or conditional independence', i.e. after the contribution of the trait to the data has been removed, all that will be left is random, normally distributed noise (Linacre 2003b). In other words, the model maintains that answers to individual items will be randomly related once the effects of the trait have been partialled out.

The scale score provided by the Rasch model is a linear function of the attribute obtained from the probabilities of individual responses.

Advantages of the Rasch model over Classical Test Theory

The Rasch model has a number of claimed advantages over Classical Test Theory in assessing patient-centred health outcomes. These are discussed briefly below. For a more comprehensive and technical account see Embretson (1996).

Rasch measures have interval properties

The Rasch model transforms item data into interval scales based on the actual empirical evidence (for an example of how this is carried out, see 'Developing a Rasch Scale' below). In contrast, the classical estimate of attribute level is not linearly related to the magnitude of the underlying trait, i.e. a Classical Test Theory (CTT) sum-scale is not an interval scale.

Item parameters and person values under Rasch/Item Response Theory are not sample-dependent, i.e. they are 'test-free'

Rasch models estimate item parameters independently of the sample employed, i.e. independently of the distribution of difficulty of the items in the sample (although how well depends on how closely the data fit the model).

In contrast, classical estimates of difficulty (e.g. 'p' or proportion correct) and discrimination (e.g. the item-total correlation), are dependent upon the pool of subjects tested. For example, an item whose 'p' value is 0.5 in a general population will have a lower value among the less able. In principle, corresponding IRT estimates do not suffer from these problems (Nunnally & Bernstein 1994, see also Hays et al 2000).

Rasch models estimate person measures independently of the items used. A Rasch/IRT model can use different sets of items for the same subject, and so allow retesting of the subject on different occasions (as memory for previous responses is not a problem). This 'test-free measurement' facilitates tailored testing and computerized adaptive testing (Nunnally & Bernstein 1994).

Rasch (1966) used the term 'specific objectivity' to describe the particular characteristic of his model which permits the comparison of two subjects independent of which instruments (stimuli) are used to measure them, as well as the comparison of two instruments independent of the subjects on whom they are used (Perline et al 1979).

Rasch/Item Response Theory models are not biased against off-target performance

Linacre (1996a) describes how the Rasch model avoids bias towards the extremes of the scale (for very high and very low scores) unlike CTT based tests. On the other hand, Rasch and True-Score validity and reliability coefficients are seen as almost identical when the trait level being assessed is in the centre of the scale (as the ogival relationship between scores and measures is close to linear).

Rasch/Item Response Theory models tolerate missing data

The Rasch model does not require a complete matrix of values as the starting point for calculations, and is 'quite robust in the face of missing data'. In contrast, classical methods require a complete data set, resulting in data having to be discarded or a substitute value placed in the missing space (Bond & Fox 2001, p. 111).

THE DIFFERENCE BETWEEN RASCH AND ITEM RESPONSE THEORY

Advocates of the Rasch model see it as *the* tool for forming measures that possess interval properties and support additivity. Specifically, measures that meet the requirements of additive conjoint measurement as formulated by Luce & Tukey (1964, see earlier in this chapter).

Those using the Rasch Model generally do so as a tool to develop interval measures, and to this end, pursue the following related features.

A focus on the measurement of a single construct

Unidimensionality in a test means that the items measure a single construct. The Rasch model is concerned to measure a single construct, with a concentration on variation in item difficulty to allow the measure to cover the range of the construct (and items of similar discrimination).

While a 2PL IRT model might better *describe* data than a Rasch model, as it allows variation in discrimination, the result is a 'highly fuzzy definition' of the latent continuum with no precise definition of what is being measured (Salzberger 2002).

Active development of a scale based on items of similar discrimination

To meet the requirements of the model, item discrimination must be constant. Rasch analysis seeks out deviations from uniform item discrimination. Guessing is similarly a threat and is sought and reported (Linacre 1999).

Note that there is never a set of items of 'equal discrimination', but the items must be of similar discrimination – both unusually low and unusually *high* discriminations require further investigation (see Masters 1993).

An emphasis on the fit of data to the model, not of the model to the data

'The Rasch model is not a data model at all. ... It's our guide to data good enough to make measures from' (Wright 1988).

Rasch Analysts seek to develop scales that avoid undesired qualities such as guessing, while IRT exponents are seen to be concerned with the descriptive power of the model. Rasch analysts are concerned to evaluate the fit of the *data to the model*, not the model to the data.

Linacre (1996b) described Rasch analysis as avoiding the incorporation of features of the data known to be sample sensitive such as guessing and discrimination, while incorporating features known to be general. He also observed that if there is little guessing and item discriminations are similar, then IRT and Rasch produce similar results; while if there are no extreme scores then raw score analysis (CTT tests) and Rasch produce similar results.

Bond & Fox (2001) describe how stress is placed upon close examination of the results of the modelling process. 'Rasch measurement works hand in hand with the investigator to determine the extent to which the data actually measure the construct under examination' (Bond & Fox 2001, p. 192).

The use of extensive quality control statistics – item maps,
fit statistics, etc.

To ensure the requirements of scientific measurement are being
met, i.e. that the data fit the Rasch model, the software used by
Rasch analysis practitioners (e.g. WINSTEPS) provides many
graphs and statistics to allow identification and scrutiny of ill-
fitting data, and hence allow decisions about which persons and
items should not remain in the model. In contrast, neither IRT nor
raw score analysis is seen to implement quality control of the construct and the data effectively (Linacre 1996b).

A willingness to commence the analysis early,
with relatively few cases

Responding to the information that 200 subjects were required for
the one parameter (Rasch) model when deriving an item characteristic curve (suggested by Streiner & Norman 1996), Wright &
Tennant (1996) stated that with a reasonably targeted sample of
50 persons there was 99% confidence that the estimated item difficulty would be close enough for most practical purposes, especially when persons take 10 or more items (within ±1 logit of its
stable value); with 200 persons, there would be 99% confidence
that the estimated value was within ±0.5 logits.

Indeed, for pilot studies, Wright & Tennant suggested that 30
persons are enough, and that analysis should begin once the first
data become available, '200 incorrect administrations are never as
good as 50 correct ones'.

Note that more cases are needed for analyzing Likert scale data
than dichotomous data. The sample needs to be varied enough so
that all the response options for all of the items are used; and with
five response options per item rather than two, proportionately
more persons are needed to achieve the same density of data for
each response (Bond & Fox 2001).

DEVELOPING A RASCH SCALE

The following indicates some of the elements of developing a
Rasch-based scale. For an understanding of the practical issues sufficient to develop a scale, further reading is needed (e.g. begin with
Bond & Fox 2001, and the extensive information accessible via
www.rasch.org). This needs to be combined with practical experience with Rasch software, such as WINSTEPS, RUMM, or QUEST.

Initial steps

The initial steps of scale development are the same for Rasch as for classical methods, i.e. clear specification of the construct to be measured, followed by development of the content, drafting and trialing of items for suitability and comprehensiveness, etc. Care should be taken to cover the range of the construct, so that items are not excessively bunched. Once the questionnaire has been administered, trial data can be analyzed and items and persons calibrated.

An example of creating a measure for the original dichotomous model is outlined in Box 8.1. Extensions of the dichotomous model have been made to handle polytomous items (items that allow more than two responses), such as the rating scale model and the partial credit model.

Box 8.1   Example: creating a measure for the dichotomous model (adapted from Bond & Fox 2001, pp. 199–200)

Bond & Fox (2001) describe the starting point as calculating the percentage correct for each person (the number of items successfully answered divided by the total number of items) and each item (the number of persons successfully passing the item divided by the total number of persons) when the test is administered to an appropriate sample. While ordinal level data, these raw scores are both necessary and sufficient for estimating person ability and item difficulty.

The first step in estimating the ability measure of a person is to convert the raw score percentage into odds of success, by calculating the ratio of each person's percentage correct (p) over the percentage incorrect (1 – p). The procedure is the same for items, estimating the difficulty measure of an item *by* dividing the percentage of people who answered the item correctly by the percentage of people who answered the item incorrectly and taking the natural log of that value.

The item difficulty and person ability estimates are then expressed on a scale of log odd ratios or logits. The average logit is arbitrarily set at 0, with positive logits indicating higher than average probabilities and negative logits indicating lower than average probabilities.

The process is an iterative one. The calculations begin by ignoring or constraining person estimates, calculating item estimates, and then using the first round of item estimates to produce a first round of person estimates. The first round of estimates then are iterated against each other to produce a parsimonious and internally consistent set of item and person parameters, so that the person ability minus item difficulty values will produce the Rasch probabilities of success.

The iteration process is said to converge when the maximum difference in item and person values during successive iterations meets a preset convergence value. This transformation turns ordinal level data (i.e. correct/incorrect responses) into interval level data for both persons and items, thereby converting descriptive, sample-dependent data into inferential measures based on probabilistic functions.

Estimating item difficulty and person ability

The results of the process of calibration are displayed in computer output as item-person maps, the estimates of person ability and item difficulty being arrayed along a logit (log odds) interval scale (Bond & Fox 2001, Linacre 2003b).

The Rasch model establishes the relative difficulty of each item stem and response category (if Likert scales). It may, for example, indicate that some Likert response categories may need to be scored differently, collapsed or reversed.

Questions can then be asked of the data, such as, 'Are the items ordered as expected?', and 'Are there enough data to provide stable estimates?'. Each person's pattern of responses can also be examined, to see if any are unexpected or inappropriate.

While Rasch analysis item-person maps usually indicate item difficulty estimates and person ability estimates, other aspects such as the precision of estimates, the fit of the items, the fit of the persons, the reliabilities of the person and item estimates, will tend to be reported in output tables.

Examining fit statistics

Analyzing the fit of the data to the Rasch model is an integral part of the process, as with any latent trait model. The fit of the data to the model is essential to develop interval item and person measures, test free item and person parameters, etc. Research into methods to assess the fit of a person's responses has been most rigorous with Rasch measurement (Smith 2000).

Once the parameters of a Rasch model are estimated, they are used to compute expected (predicted) response patterns on each item. Fit statistics are then derived from a comparison of the expected patterns and the observed patterns. These fit statistics are used as a measure of the validity of the model-data fit and as a diagnosis of individual idiosyncrasy (Lusardi & Smith 1997).

Smith (2000) states that it is possible to think of the results of a test administration in two ways. The first is based on the observed score matrix, and the second on the expected score for each person on every item based on a latent trait model. Smith describes the Pearsonian chi-square approach to estimating fit, observing that the difference between the observed data and the expected results may be calculated to form a score residual matrix. Three common fits tested are then:

- overall fit of the data to the model (sum over the entire data matrix)
- the fit of the responses to a particular item, or item fit (summing across persons)
- fit of the responses by a particular person, or person fit (sum across items).

For further discussion and explanation see Smith (2000).

Item fit and person fit statistics

Item fit statistics are used to verify the internal validities of the items in contributing to a unitary scale. The model requires that an item has a greater probability of yielding a higher rating for persons with higher ability than for persons with lower ability. Those items identified as not fitting the Rasch model need to be examined and either revised or eliminated. Such an item may not be related to the rest of the scale; it may assess a different concept to that shared by the other items (Lusardi & Smith 1997).

Person fit statistics measure the extent to which a person's pattern of responses to the items correspond to that predicted by the model. A valid response, as specified by the model, dictates that a person of a given ability has a greater probability of providing a higher rating on easier items than on more difficult items. Persons identified as misfitting may not be from the targeted sample or the content of the assessment may not be appropriate for the given person (Lusardi & Smith 1997).

Cella & Chang (2000) observed that evidence of person misfit can provide valuable diagnostic information in the clinical setting.

Infit and outfit

Infit refers to inlier-sensitive or information-weighted fit. Infit is sensitive to unexpected responses to items near a person's ability level (Lusardi & Smith 1997). Linacre (2002) describes this as more sensitive to the pattern of responses to items targeted on the person. *Outfit* means outlier-sensitive fit. Outfit is sensitive to aberrant behaviour on items far from a person's ability level (Lusardi & Smith 1997). For example, outfit reports underfit for lucky guesses and careless mistakes (Linacre 2002). Items or persons with fit statistics outside

-2 to $+2$ range need to be evaluated (Lusardi & Smith 1997). For further discussion of fit statistics, see Smith (2000) and Linacre (2002).

Reliability

Linacre (2003b) states that in Rasch terms, classical 'test reliability' is an estimate of 'true person variance/observed person variance' for the particular sample of persons on the particular set of test items. Thus it is a 'person sample reliability' rather than a 'test reliability', where reliability is reproducibility of person ordering. For further information on the relationship between raw-score-based reliability (classical reliability) and measure-based reliability (Rasch reliability), see Linacre (1997).

The Rasch model provides both person and item reliabilities. The *person reliability index* indicates the degree to which the same ordering of persons would be expected if the same persons were given another set of items measuring the same construct, while the *item reliability index* indicates the degree to which the same relative item locations would be expected if the same items were given another sample of persons with similar ability levels (Bond & Fox 2001, pp. 31, 32).

Note that Rasch software such as WINSTEPS also provide classical Cronbach Alpha/KR-20 statistics, based on the raw scores (see Linacre 2003b).

Removal of items and persons to achieve adequate fit

Reflecting the Rasch focus on fit to the model, items and persons may be removed and the scale re-calibrated until an adequate fit is reached. Linacre (1999) observed that if the ideal fit is pursued, this process could conceivably continue until all are removed (the Rasch model is seen as an unreachable ideal and no data ever fit it perfectly). Instead, the iterative procedure of removing items or persons should stop when the measures are adequate for their purposes.

Note that in some cases, instead of removing problem items it may be better to reword them (or modify or condense the response categories; Bond & Fox 2001).

In this respect, Smith (2000) states that common sense is necessary in interpreting fit statistics, and that, not only the magnitude of the fit statistics should be considered, but also the standardized residuals on which the fit statistics are based. Smith gave the example of an item that misfits when taken by 100 persons, observing that if the standardized residuals indicate that most of the misfit is coming from three low ability persons who happened to get the item correct, it is probably better to keep the item ('it might be best not to drop an item that works for 97% of the sample, no matter how inappropriate it is for those three persons'; Smith 2000, p. 216).

ASSESSING MULTIDIMENSIONALITY

The successful application of Rasch analysis depends on the items representing the targeted dimension. However, where several dimensions are strongly represented in the data, the fit statistics may be inadequate. Identifying multidimensionality may require both Rasch analysis and factor analysis.

The evidence is that Rasch analysis based on fit statistics alone, can produce misleading results. As described by Linacre (1998), Rasch analysis constructs an interval variable from the dominant dimension (factor) in the data. This dominant dimension may be a hybrid (e.g. if a test has both mobility and depression items, the dominant factor may be a composite of mobility-depression), with lesser dimensions reported as misfit. Several simulation studies have indicated that Rasch fit statistics can be insensitive to multidimensionality, in both the Rasch dichotomous and rating scale model (Smith 1996, Smith & Miao 1994). This may apply where there are approximately equal numbers of items on each factor, such as a functional assessment inventory that contains 8 motor skills items and 8 cognitive items (Smith 2000, see also Wright 1996). Because of this, it generally recommended that principal component analysis of the item scores or the Rasch residuals is also conducted.

Should principal components analysis be applied to raw scores or Rasch residuals?

Rasch analysis may be preceded by the application of Principal Components Analysis (PCA) to the raw scores to distinguish the first factor, with the corresponding items then analyzed via the Rasch model. McHorney et al (2000) recommended that to determine unidimensionality, PCA should first be conducted, with any items correlating less than 0.4 with the first un-rotated principal component to be removed as well as any items correlating substantially with multiple components (as they do not contribute to just one health construct).

However, Linacre (1998) argued that factor analysis of raw scores (the original observations) is likely to be misleading, as:

- the observations are non-linear and can generate illusory factors; and
- factor analysis can report items clustering at different performance levels as different factors.

This suggests that PCA should be applied to the Rasch residuals, not the raw scores (Linacre 1998, Schumacker & Linacre 1996). Smith (2002) reported further simulation and empirical data in support of this. Wright (1996) can be consulted for an example of applying PCA to Rasch residuals with the Functional Independence Measure (FIM-SM) instrument.

Note that the presence of Rasch residual variance does not mean that the data is not to all extents and purposes unidimensional; Smith & Miao (1994) found by simulation that 'perfect' Rasch data produced small residual factors.

Estimating values

Rasch software provides estimated measures and standard errors for all possible scores on the test, along with a graph of the score to measure conversion (Linacre 2003b). This information can be used to form self-scoring maps for data recording, estimating ability, normative comparison, etc. Linacre (1995) illustrated this with the 'KeyFIM', a redesigned form used for data collection and immediate feedback of measurement and diagnostic analysis when using the FIM-SM to assess patient rehabilitation.

APPLICATIONS OF RASCH/ITEM RESPONSE THEORY IN HEALTH OUTCOMES MEASUREMENT

Improving/assessing existing tests and developing new ones

There is growing evidence that Rasch analysis/IRT can increase the ability of existing tests to detect health outcome effects.

Raczek et al (1998) compared the current Likert scoring method of the SF-36 physical functioning scale (PF-10) with scoring algorithms based on the Rasch model in general population respondents in Denmark, Germany, Italy, the Netherlands, Sweden, the UK and the USA. They found Rasch scoring methods to be superior in discriminating among age groups in all countries, and it was concluded that Rasch models hold good potential for improving health status measures, estimating individual scores when responses to scale items are missing, and equating scores across countries.

Birbeck et al (2000) evaluated the ability of HQoL measures to detect change over time in persons with epilepsy. Using two different criteria for change (one based on seizure frequency, one on self-reported overall condition), they compared responsiveness for the SF-36 (using the current scoring method and a Rand-36 method based on IRT), the SF-12, and two epilepsy-targeted HQoL measures. Birbeck et al found that while the two epilepsy-specific measures in general had the larger responsiveness indices, the IRT-based responsiveness indices were comparable to the epilepsy-specific measures for the criterion of change in seizure frequency. Moreover, the IRT-based scoring system was superior to the traditional scoring of the SF-36, which revealed less sensitivity to change, with the SF-12 responsiveness indices smaller again. Birbeck et al concluded that the IRT scoring method increased the instrument's validity.

IRT methods have also been employed to identify subjects for whom a test is unsuitable. Schmitt et al (1999) applied the two-parameter logistic model implemented in the BILOG programme to examine the consistency of individuals' response patterns with their estimated trait levels on cognitive ability and personality tests (e.g. individuals with high estimates as measured by a test would be considered not to fit the IRT model if they provided substantial numbers of incorrect responses to items of low difficulty). Schmitt et al concluded that person misfit was present and may be related to gender and race.

There is a growing number of new tests being developed to measure health outcomes that include Rasch methods; for example, Leplège et al (1997) measuring quality of life (QoL) from the point of view of human immunodeficiency virus (HIV)-positive subjects, and Badia et al (2002) with the development of the Osteoporosis-Specific Quality of Life Questionnaire.

Item banking and computer adaptive testing

Because Rasch/IRT reveals the response characteristics of individual items and the relationships between individual items, it is possible to set up pre-calibrated stores of items classified by HQoL domain that can then be used to construct more efficient scales (Revicki & Cella 1997). For example, Badia et al (2002) describe the use of IRT to form a new, more efficient scale for measuring osteoporosis HQoL from two pre-existing scales.

Item banks

Collections of calibrated items form item banks, 'collections of test items coded by subject area etc. and various item characteristics such as item difficulty and discrimination' (Rudner 1998). Using an IRT method such as the Rasch model, items from multiple tests can be placed on a common scale, the scale indicating the relative difficulty of the items. New tests with predictable characteristics can then be developed by drawing items from the bank.

McHorney & Cohen (2000) reported locating more than 75 instruments available to measure functional status (differing in number of items, type of rating scale, and item difficulty). They described their application of IRT to calibrate a large number of these items on the same scale, to allow a better understanding of the structure, order, and interrelationships between functional status items. Revicki & Cella (1997) described the use of item banks to establish large sets of questions representing various levels of a HQoL domain, that can then be used to develop brief, efficient scales for measuring the domain.

Computer adaptive testing

In computer adaptive testing (CAT), the difficulty of test items administered is specifically tailored to the ability level of the test taker, so as to provide an individualized examination. CAT operates on the principle that items that are too easy or too difficult for the candidate contribute little information about the test taker's ability. Thus on-target information is maximized (i.e. the items more correspond to the ability level of the testee), the standard error of measurement (SEM) is minimized and the test can be much shorter without sacrificing reliability (Bond & Fox 2001).

CAT can entail the application of IRT and item banks to provide tailored assessments of HQoL domains specific to individual patients. This allows more efficient and brief scales to measure multiple domains of HQoL, and to measure HQoL across different stages of disease (Revicki & Cella 1997). See also Uttaro & Lehman (1999) and Ware et al (2000).

Identifying item bias in diverse patient groups

A major area of concern is item bias or differential item functioning (DIF). DIF is where item parameters vary across groups, i.e. an item varies in difficulty or discrimination from one group to another. To the extent that this occurs, tests will provide misleading results.

Linacre (1996b) noted that constant item parameters imply a constant construct, and different item parameters across samples of the relevant population imply the construct has changed. The result is that measures can not be compared across samples. Rasch analysis specifies that item parameters be sample independent, and provides methods for investigating where and by how much, different samples fail to conform to this principle of measurement.

CTT has the shortcoming that the values of the parameters of the test items (item difficulty and item discrimination) depend on the particular sample to whom the items are administered (although there are CTT approaches for investigating DIF, e.g. see Nunnally & Bernstein 1994). In contrast, the item parameters obtained using IRT are claimed to be independent of the sample tested. If a given item is unbiased, then the estimated ICCs for that item should be the same for the different groups examined. Rasch/IRT software provides detailed item- and person-level information to identify items that exhibit DIF.

Both unusually low and unusually high discriminations need investigation. Masters (1993) gives the example of a second language listening comprehension test in German, where test results for native and non-native speakers revealed an unusually discriminating item. Investigation showed the item concerned German politics (native-speaking students would have an advantage because of their ordinary knowledge of German politics). The item was highly discriminating because of its sensitivity to a second dimension that was highly correlated with the variable of interest (it was deleted).

In the context of health, Cella & Chang (2000) observed that the hererogeneity of patient populations may mean that item parameters will vary across different patient groups. Item bias needs to be investigated comprehensively.

For further discussion of item bias under Rasch, see Smith (1992).

Test equating

Test equating is conducted after tests have been constructed to provide a common scale for attribute/ability estimates. Rasch/ IRT models offer significant advantages in test equating over CTT given their ability to identify item bias. Two types of equating are:

• Horizontal equating, which requires the development of a common metric for a pool of items or tests intended to measure individuals with similar levels of the attribute/ability, e.g. tests that are designed to assess HQoL for those with the same or similar medical condition (such as osteoporosis, see Badia et al 2002).
• Vertical equating, which requires the development of a common metric for a pool of items or tests designed to measure individuals with markedly different levels of the attribute/ ability (possibly for individuals with the same illness but at different ends of the disease process, such as in HIV).

If the tests have been formed from Rasch calibrated item banks, there is seen to be no need to conduct test equating, since the tests will already be in the common logit metric (Smith 1992).

For further information, see Smith (1992) and Bond & Fox (2001).

RASCH AND TESTS BASED ON MULTIPLE DIMENSIONS

Most tests and test models are targeted at measuring a single dimension. Each of the common scale types, i.e. CTT/Likert, Thurstone's Method of Equal-appearing Intervals, Guttman, and Rasch analysis, entail unidimensional scaling methods.

On the face of it this would seem a problem for the measurement of a construct such as HQoL where its nature as 'multidimensional' is almost universally asserted.

Three different approaches that Rasch users might take to this issue are considered here.

1. Maintain that all scales are unidimensional, including HQoL

A 'unidimensional scale' measures a single dimension or concept using a single number. On the other hand 'multidimensional

HQoL' refers to QoL being influenced by a broad range of different factors, each of which corresponds to a 'construct' or 'dimension'. However, HQoL can also be a superordinate dimension, expressed in the patient's reply to the question, 'How do you rate your quality of life on a scale of 1–10?'. The patient may be influenced by a number of different issues in providing a response, but a meaningful answer is generally forthcoming.

Dimensions, or constructs, are in the eye of the beholder. Stahl (1990) argued that in considering what is a 'dimension' statistical arguments are not useful, for it is the intention of the questioner or researcher that defines the dimension.

Moreover, when a construct is developed that defines a dimension, the potential for establishing hierarchies of dimensions is opened, with one researcher's multidimensional space being another researcher's unidimensional line of concern: there could be a unidimensional operationalization of the entire field of mathematics, and at the same time algebra and geometry could each be a single dimension. Anything can be defined as unidimensional. As Stahl puts it, 'It is useful to think of unidimensionality not as an opportune empirical accident but rather as an intended theoretical construct to be defined. The intention of the researcher must be explicit. What is the construct to be measured?'

As expressed by Wright (1994), 'we use our imaginations to invent a construct … [Wright gives the example of math ability] … that suits our purposes. This construct is our dimension'.

However, there is a responsibility that the thinking and logic needed to establish the intended construct and its relationship to other variables is executed thoroughly. Rasch analysis attempts to form a scale from the variance that most of the items share – the analysis is blind to whether this first factor is or is not the one being aimed at by the test developer.

Stenner (2001) observes that it is easy to apply the Rasch model without a construct theory, that Rasch programmes enable practitioners to estimate item difficulties and person measures on a logit or transformed logit scale, but to be scientific, enough should be known about the construct to be able to specify item calibrations prior to data collection (otherwise Rasch will be like exploratory factor analysis, 'producing too many successful studies').

2. Accept 'some multidimensionality' within a primarily unidimensional scale

There are those who have identified multidimensionality in a scale and ignored it. This particularly applies with pre-existing scales that were not developed to be Rasch measures, but where Rasch techniques are applied 'after the event' to improve the validity of the instrument: offering an alternative scoring method is presumably much more practically acceptable to existing users than changing the items.

For example, Wolfe & Kong (1999) investigated the extent to which the Western Ontario MacMaster osteoarthritis questionnaire (WOMAC) satisfied the Rasch model, particularly regarding unidimensionality, item separation, and linearity. The Winsteps programme was applied, with the result that several functional items were found to have a high information weight fit statistic (INFIT; see Linacre 2003a, b), indicating poor fit to the model. These items included 'getting in and out of the bath' and 'going down stairs'.

Wolfe & Kong concluded that removing such items would have little effect on the model overall, and it would be difficult to remove these traces of multidimensionality while keeping the central constructs of progressive lower body musculoskeletal abnormality intact. It was felt that a 'purer' more unidimensional instrument would be less useful in clinical trials and epidemiological studies by restricting the range of the scale. See also Tsuji et al (2000).

Another example is the view argued by Linacre (1996b), in opposing Dickson & Kohler (1996). Dickson & Kohler reported finding that a unidimensional construct did not underlie the motor items of the Functional Independence Measure (FIM), and Rasch analysis would not lead to interval properties in their measurement. They stated that, 'The principal components analysis shows that for all impairment groups ... the dimensionality is at least six. To explain 80% of the variance three factors are required.' In reply to this, Linacre (1996b) pointed out that while the motor FIM was unidimensional for 'practical purposes', it was true there was some degree of multidimensionality in the data: the second factor identified in Dickson & Kohler's analysis was dominated by 'bowel' and 'bladder', which were known to misfit the motor scale due to their socio-emotional aspects but 'are kept in the measurement system due their clinical importance'.

3.   Develop multiple Rasch scales and combine them

While there is little evidence of tests that combine Rasch-based unidimensional subscales to produce overall test scores, they are likely to have merit.

Following from the previous section, Dickson & Kohler (1996) observed that the item order Rasch analysis produced in motor FIM data was simplistic. For example, climbing stairs was placed as more difficult than eating, yet Dickson & Kohler observed, 'we have seen people who could ... climb stairs, but not swallow. These patients do not fit the interval scale'.

The response of Linacre (1996b) was that the Rasch model is a theoretical ideal, a definition of measurement, and the relevant question was, 'Do the items fit the Rasch model well enough to construct useful measures?' Moreover, such data (cannot eat but can climb stairs) were only *very unexpected* with a Rasch-constructed interval scale, and would be predicted to occur occasionally (being a probabilistic model).

While Linacre's view is defensible, it is apparent that in modelling the motor data, the best fit was one that could lead to a disadvantage for some patient groups, such as those with throat problems. (It would depend on the purpose to which the test was put; as emphasized in Ch. 4, tests are not valid per se, *applications* are more or less valid.)

One could argue that health-related conditions may be *particularly* unsuitable for omnibus unidimensional Rasch HQoL scales, given that incapacities can occur throughout the body in varying intensities, and for accidents, might even be considered random (as opposed to, say, items that reflect a developmental series or its inverse, as are common in education).

A similar issue was raised by Cella & Chang (2000). They queried a suggestion by McHorney & Cohen (2000) that items measuring long-distance travel could be added to items assessing short-term memory to measure functional status. Cella & Chang suggested that this raised a question about the fit of items with one another along the dimension being measured. If a clinically heterogeneous mixture of questions could indeed be scaled as a unidimensional construct (as was the Dickson & Kohler FIM example), what would the construct mean?

There are other ways of using the benefits of Rasch analysis in measuring complex constructs, such as to separate the various attributes/factors that are related to overall HQoL into their own Rasch dimensions. Consistent with such a proposal, Linacre (1996b) observed that, 'Usually, if the data have any meaning at all, they can be segmented into meaningful subsets that do fit the Rasch model and do support inference', and indicated support for an approach that explicitly took into account criterion validity observing that, 'if it is discovered that Item 5 ... is particularly highly correlated with an indicator variable, then ... constructing measures based on a test of items like Item 5 may be useful'.

Anastasi (1990) considered this same question in the context of CTT theory, recognizing that external validation and internal consistency (or in this context, Rasch measurement) were both desirable objectives of test construction. The relative emphasis to be placed on each was dependent on the nature and purpose of the test. Anastasi proposed that where this was a dilemma, a resolution was to develop homogeneity (in the current context, Rasch properties) within sub-tests, and criterion validity across sub-tests (allowing heterogeneity).

In other words, to develop a means of estimating HQoL that can be applied to a range of different health conditions, one might form multiple Rasch sub-tests corresponding to different attributes to provide interval measures of each (e.g.'eating', 'walking', 'cognitive ability', etc.). The validity of the overall test (battery of sub-tests) would be developed by combining sub-test scores to predict a criterion. The criterion might be global patient report using a visual analogue scale (VAS), and the VAS could itself be transformed into a Rasch scale before being used to combine the sub-tests (see Thomee et al 1995).

In conclusion, it may be better to form multiple Rasch unidimensional sub-tests of factors relevant to HQoL, with the subscales then combined to form an omnibus HQoL estimate where necessary.

There are potentially a range of ways of effecting the combination, from a discount function (see Ch. 2 under 'The Global Evaluation of an Experienced State Is Not the Sum of Its Parts', and Ch. 7 under 'Developing a Method for Combining Sub-test Scores'), to the use of VAS-derived anchors based on observed relationships to each sub-test. The issue is an empirical one.

SUMMARY

*Should measures of psychological attributes have interval
properties?*

The statistical view – measures of constructs do not need interval
properties:

- Psychological scales may not have interval properties, but
  they may quite justifiably be treated as if they have interval or
  ratio properties for statistical purposes.

The 'representational' view – measures of constructs can, and
should, have interval properties:

- The Rasch psychometric model, a practical expression of
  conjoint additivity, can provide an additive framework and
  measures with interval properties.

At the coal face:

- Ignoring interval properties leads to perceptibly poor items.

Latent trait models: IRT and the Rasch model

ICCs:

- The ICC relates the probability of a response to an item to the
  strength of an underlying trait.
- The model is probabilistic. The likelihood of the item being
  affirmed is indicated by the difficulty and discrimination of
  the item, as well as the ability (strength of attribute) of the
  person.
- The ICC is typically assumed to be a logistic ogive.

The latent trait family:

- The one-parameter logistic model and the Rasch model
  assume that items vary only with respect to their difficulty,
  i.e. all have the same discrimination, and they cannot be
  answered correctly by guessing.
- In other IRT models, items vary in discrimination and/or
  guessing also.

The Rasch model

The probability of a person getting a correct response on an item is a function of the difference between a person's ability and an item's difficulty. When there is a fit of the Rasch model, items and persons are measured on a common interval scale.

Advantages of the Rasch model over CTT:

- Rasch measures have interval properties.
- Rasch/IRT item parameters are not sample-dependent (i.e. are test-free).
- test-free person values.
- Rasch/IRT models are not biased against off-target performance.
- Rasch/IRT models tolerate missing data.

The difference between Rasch and IRT:

- a focus on the measurement of a single construct.
- active development of a scale based on items of similar discrimination.
- an emphasis on the fit of data to the model, not of the model to the data.
- the use of extensive quality control statistics – item maps, fit statistics, etc.
- a willingness to commence the analysis early, with relatively few cases.

Developing a Rasch scale:

- the initial steps are the same for Rasch as for developing a good classical test.
- after the questionnaire has been administered the data are analyzed to calculate parameters for items and persons.
- the estimates of person ability and item difficulty are arrayed along a logit (log odds) interval scale.
- the fit of the data to the Rasch model is examined.
- the Rasch model provides both person and item reliabilities.
- items and persons may be removed and the scale re-calibrated until an adequate fit is reached.
- identifying multidimensionality may require both Rasch analysis and factor analysis.

- Rasch software provides estimated measures and standard errors for all possible scores on the test, along with a graph of the score to measure conversion.

Applications of Rasch/IRT in health outcomes measurement:

- improving/assessing existing tests and developing new ones
- item Banking and Computer Adaptive Testing
- identifying item bias in diverse patient groups
- test equating.

Rasch and tests based on multiple dimensions

Approaches to measuring a 'multidimensional' construct:

- maintain that all scales are unidimensional, including HQoL
- accept 'some multi-dimensionality' within a primarily unidimensional scale
- develop multiple Rasch scales and combine them where necessary.

CONCLUDING POINTS

- Rasch analysis and IRT only consider part of the test construction process. As with any test, the most important part is a clear definition of what is to be tested, the inclusion of demonstrably necessary and sufficient content, and following development, evidence that the results meet suitable external criteria.
- Second, most tests that are well formed by CTT standards will probably perform acceptably. In this respect, Linacre (1999) observed that since the central part of the ogival model ICC is almost straight, a high correlation is expected between measures and raw scores for complete on-target response patterns, but that raw score analysis (CTT) deals badly with broader targeting, missing data, incoherent response patterns and test equating.
- Fan (1998) empirically examined the behaviour of item and person parameters obtained from the CTT and IRT measurement frameworks with very large samples. The findings were that the

two measurement frameworks produced very similar item and person statistics (however, the fit of the data for the Rasch model was poor, with about 30% of the items identified as misfitting, so the results via a better Rasch model are unknown).

- Third, while Rasch/IRT based tests are likely to be superior (although care seems to be needed when advocates try to shoe-horn diverse items into a unidimensional model), they demand a much greater degree of sophistication from the test developer. As observed by Nunnally & Bernstein (1994), the classical test model is much simpler and may be sufficient in the vast majority of applications, and suggested that someone who is not well versed in psychometric theory begin by constructing a test classically (they also suggested that proponents of IRT tend to exaggerate the role of statistical inference over description).

  The application of Rasch analysis (and IRT) requires the use of theory and algorithms that are more complex than CTT, applied via software that at the time of writing this book was complex and not user-friendly. As a result, users could be tempted to take a 'black-box approach' and develop overly simplified and invalid models. This particularly applies when dealing with highly diverse items ('multidimensional data').

  Clancy & Lipscomb (2000) suggested that new approaches based on IRT offer potential, but the tradeoffs in moving from classic psychometric approaches have not been fully explored.

- Fourth, there remains the need to stress the criterion validity of measures. There is a sense in which Rasch/IRT, like CTT, can be 'begging the question'; that is, assuming that the items modelled are representing the construct that is being targeted. Notwithstanding the stress placed on testing fit and examining residuals, etc. Rasch analysis could conceivably create a dimension out of multiple constructs, leading to the illusion that one is assessing a single construct when it is actually a composite. Both CTT and Rasch may ignore predictive validity; both *assume* the items are measuring the right thing. In patient-centred health outcomes measurement, the ability to predict the criterion of patient self-assessed HQoL should also be considered.

  Reliance on internal properties of tests is no substitute for external demonstrations of validity. In Rasch/IRT and classical methods, there is the need for clarity regarding what is really meant by validity – the purpose of the measure and the constructs being assessed (see Chs 3 and 4). Just as with CTT, testing of the ability of the test to predict meaningful external events (a criterion variable such as self-assessed HQoL or seizure frequency) is essential.

- Fifth, as noted by Cella & Chang (2000), Rasch/IRT was originally developed for and used with a fairly homogeneous educational assessment population. In health, these methods are likely to be applied to more heterogeneous clinical populations. Items are likely to mean different things in different populations (i.e. DIF). Having to deal with what must be almost the most heterogeneous of all areas, HQoL, possibly encompassing patient-subjective and objective elements, offers different issues and challenges.
- Finally, Rasch/IRT provides a way to answer real concerns that CTT testers have consistently failed to address. It also requires the user to think about what they are doing. The challenge is to understand and apply Rasch/IRT while realizing that it is likely to be part of the answer, but not all of it.

QUOTABLE QUOTE

All the IRT in the world will not save a bad test.
(Nunnally & Bernstein 1994, p. 442)

A great deal of information on Rasch test development is available through the Institute for Objective Measurement and its extensive set of links to papers, links to software (e.g. WINSTEPS, QUEST, RUMM) and internet forums. See www.rasch.org. The Rasch community is vibrant, active, and highly supportive. *The Journal of Applied Measurement* is largely dedicated to the Rasch model and the development of interval measures.

The development of some generic instruments

AIMS OF CHAPTER

- To indicate the widely varying nature of tests

- To give examples of the way tests originate

- To illustrate some different test development forms

The following reviews the development of some prominent health status assessment tools. The accounts are focussed on the steps involved in developing the instruments, not on their most recent configurations or applications.

SICKNESS IMPACT PROFILE

The Sickness Impact Profile (SIP) was originally developed by Bergner and co-workers, as part of funding from the US National Center for Health Service Research to develop general measures of health status (Bergner et al 1976a, Bergner et al 1976b). The SIP, Quality of Well-Being index (QWB), and the General Health Rating Index later developed by the Rand Corporation to become the Rand Health Status Measure, were all results of this initiative.

Kaplan et al (1989) noted that each of these measures was 'guided by the WHO definition of health status: 'Health is a complete state of physical, mental and social well-being and not merely absence of disease' (Kaplan et al 1989, p. S31).

The SIP was developed with the specific aim of providing information on the efficacy of health programmes to assist decisions regarding the appropriate allocation of the government's resources. It was aimed to provide a 'fiscally and logistically practical measure of health status' (Bergner et al 1976a, p. 393).

In developing their measure, Bergner et al referred to three broad conceptions of health on which individuals base their appraisal of their own health status (Barmann 1961, cited in Bergner et al 1976a). These were a feeling state conception, a clinical conception, and a performance conception. Feeling state refers to statements of the type, 'I feel good', or 'I don't feel well today'. Clinical conception refers to specific symptoms, and performance conception refers to activities that can or cannot be performed.

Bergner et al decided that only the last of these, the performance conception, was suitable. It could be based on respondent report, but could also be easily observed and reported by an untrained observer, and also allowed easy comparison between different diseases and dysfunctions. The feeling state conception was ruled out as it is seen to be inaccessible to external validation, and the clinical conception was seen as unsuitable as it required medical interpretation and hence was reliant on the definitions of physicians and not the person concerned.

The SIP was hence conceptualized as *'an instrument which would provide a descriptive profile of the responses of a given individual in terms of the specific behavioural impacts of sickness'* (Bergner et al 1976a, p. 401), with the impacts capable of being summarized within specific areas of living as well as in some form of overall assessment.

Box 9.1 Examples of items from the Sickness Impact Profile (SIP)

Subjects are to indicate the items that describe them on the day of testing and are related to their health. There are 136 items (in 12 categories). For example:

I am going out less to visit people (social interaction)
I am not going into town (mobility)
I act nervously or restlessly (emotional behaviour)

(Examples from Damiano 1996)

Initial development

Item preparation

The instrument was developed by first preparing a list of health-related dysfunctions that would cover a range from minimal to maximal dysfunction. These were obtained from patients, healthcare professionals, individuals caring for patients, and the apparently healthy. From this process was obtained 1100 statements describing a dysfunction and the corresponding behaviour. Through a process of refinement, the SIP instrument was reduced to 312 items in 14 categories.

The items were simple, first person statements in the present tense, of the type that appear in attitude scales. The categories included areas such as social interaction e.g. 'I am going out less to visit people'; mobility and confinement, e.g. 'I stay within my room'; emotion, feelings, and sensations, e.g. 'I act nervously or restlessly'. The items were to be administered by trained interviewers, and the respondents were to respond only to items that they were sure described themselves on the day, and that were related to their health.

Single-item scaling

The items were scaled by asking judges to allocate each item within a category to an 11-point scale, ranging from minimally to severely dysfunctional. The most and least dysfunctional items from each category were then allocated to a 15-point scale, with the intra-category items then re-scaled mathematically to ensure consistency across categories.

Item and judge reliability-testing

The judges were seven nursing students, eight medical students, four physicians, and six health administration students. T-tests showed no significant differences between the clinically sophisticated and unsophisticated types of judges in terms of mean scale values measured per item.

Items scaled by different judges such that their 95% confidence intervals were more than 2 scale points apart were deleted (29 of the initial 312 items).

Item combinations

The development steps described so far were concerned to scale individual items. However, patients would normally possess numbers of items (item profiles) and to adjust for item interactions, 246 patients were assessed for the applicability of each item. Further groups of judges were then used to make global ratings of dysfunction of each subject's protocol of responses in each category of the SIP, and to then rate each subject's complete SIP on a 15-point scale.

Four methods of scoring the SIP profiles were considered, including a mean of the scale values used, a mean of the squared values (i.e. weights high scoring items), percent of total possible dysfunction (total of scored items/total possible score × 100), and a profile, the number of items checked in each of four groupings, where groupings were determined by the values of the items. Thus, items of value 15–11 were in group 1, 10–7 in group 2, 6–5 in group 3, and 4–1 in group 4. A profile of 1430 would mean 0 scores between 1 and 4, 3 scores between 5 and 6, 4 of between 7 and 10, and 1 between 11 and 15.

Correlations between scoring methods and global ratings were conducted to determine which were most suitable. The results were that the profile and percent methods gave the highest correlations with the global assessments, and Bergner et al suggested that the protocol judges appeared to attend to both the number of items checked and the items checked with the highest value (although they did not know the item scale values).

Further work was carried out to validate the instrument, e.g. using multiple regression analyses to look at interrelationships between items when used to describe subjects. Regression analyses were conducted separately for groups of subjects whose SIPs were rated as 'high dysfunction' and those rated as 'low dysfunction'. These analyses were made to ensure that items that were useful predictors for severe or minimally dysfunctional subjects, but that were not useful predictors for the sample as a whole, were retained in the revised SIP.

Bergner et al noted that the SIP was designed to assess health-related dysfunction as opposed to quality of life (QoL), and was not intended to be used as a sole criterion for either evaluating health programmes or assessing population health levels.

1974 field validation

Bergner et al (1976b) reported on the field validation of a 1974 version of the SIP, using a 235 item version of the SIP.

This and later versions employed a scaling system where a SIP percent score was calculated by summing the scale values of items checked, and dividing by the sum of the scale values for all items, and multiplying by 100. Such scores may be calculated for the whole SIP (all items) and individual categories.

To validate the SIP against a field population, 278 subjects were gathered in four sub-samples: rehabilitation medicine patients, speech pathology patients, out-patients with chronic problems, and group practice attenders. The SIP scores on these patients were compared to subjects' self-assessments of both sickness and general dysfunction, clinicians' assessments for the out-patients and speech pathology patients, and scores on the functional assessment instruments of the activities of daily living (ADL) scale and NHIS (National Health Interview Survey, providing a gross estimate of functional restriction in the previous 2 weeks).

It should be noted that the self-assessment instructions differed by more than concerning sickness/injury or poor functioning: the function instructions were much longer, more detailed, described the way in which functioning could be diminished, and as a product were also less ambiguous.

Discriminant capacity

The four sub-sample groups were analyzed using analysis of variance (ANOVA), revealing a significant main effect of group, i.e. patient type influenced SIP score as would be expected given the differences between the groups.

Self-assessment of health status

For the whole sample, the correlation (r) between self-assessment scores and SIP scores was moderately high and significant (for self-assessed sickness $r = 0.54$ and for self-assessed dysfunction $r = 0.52$), but there was a trend for correlations to be higher for some sub-samples. Thus for group practice patients, the correlation coefficients were $r = 0.74$ and 0.45, for chronic patients $r = 0.37$ and 0.42, and for speech pathology patients $r = 0.21$ and -0.1 (non-significant). SIP scores that best predicted the self-assessments were determined using multiple regression, revealing that four of the categories (ambulation, mobility and confinement, body movement, leisure pastimes) were most highly related to self-assessment scores.

Clinical assessments

The SIP scores for chronic patients correlated 0.49 (p < 0.001) with clinical rating, although it was noteworthy that the strength of the correlation declined with the length of time in practice. For these physicians the SIP categories of ambulation, mobility and confinement, and sleep and rest behaviour were most predictive of their rating. The SIP score for speech pathology patients correlated non-significantly with the ratings of their clinicians.

Relationships between self-assessment and clinician assessment

The correlation between chronic patients' self-assessments and their clinicians' assessments was moderately high and significant (r = 0.52, p < 0.001). However, the corresponding correlation for speech pathology patients was low and non-significant.

This data showed again how an overall moderate or high correlation may mask shortcomings in sensitivity for particular subgroups. For example, the correlation for the total sample between self-assessment of dysfunction and SIP score was 0.52. This was more than each of the sub-groups alone, with the correlation for speech pathology patients being −0.01.

Assessment based on activities of daily living and the National Health Interview Survey

SIP correlated with the ADL score for rehabilitation patients 0.46 (p < 0.01), while the NHIS correlated with SIP for all patients 0.61 (p < 0.001). However, again, the aggregate score masked major lack of sensitivity for some groups. Thus rehabilitation patients correlated only 0.17 (non-significant) and speech pathology patients 0.30 (non-significant), versus chronic patients 0.52 (p < 0.001) and group practice patients 0.58 (p < 0.001).

> These SIP data demonstrate the importance for the validation of health status instruments to closely examine different patient populations, and to use a range of convergent and discriminant measures.

1976 field testing

As described by Bergner et al (1981), the final form of the SIP followed a 1976 field testing, entailing study of a large structured random sample from a prepaid group practice, plus a quota of self-described sick people from a family medicine clinic. The field testing resulted in the SIP being reduced to 136 statements in 12 areas of activity, with the final form of the instrument capable of being administered in 20 to 30 minutes, or of being self-administered. It covered physical dysfunction, psychosocial dysfunction, and a number of independent areas such as eating, work, sleep and rest, etc.

Administration mode

As part of the 1976 field testing, Bergner et al investigated the reliability of three types of administration: interviewer administered; interviewer delivered and explained and then self-administered; and mail delivered and self-administered. It was found that mail-delivered, self-administered SIPs had the lowest internal consistency reliability (measured by Cronbach's Alpha), and also the lowest correlations with self-assessed dysfunction and illness. In fact, the interviewer-delivered and explained and then self-administered mode produced the greatest correlations with self-assessment dysfunction and illness scores, these being 0.74 and 0.67 correspondingly, vs correlations of 0.64 and 0.55 for interviewer-administered, and 0.48 and 0.38 for mail-delivered.

Convergent/discriminant validity

The validity of the SIP was again assessed, with tests of its ability to correlate highly with overall self-assessment, and to correlate less highly with overall clinicians' assessment and other instruments.

SIP scores were found to be most correlated with self-assessment of dysfunction (0.69), followed by self-assessment of sickness (0.63), then NHIS index (0.55), and least correlated with clinicians assessment of illness (0.40). This pattern of diminishing correlations was seen to be consistent with the construct as planned.

Correlations were further examined within a model similar to the multitrait-multimethod technique of Campbell & Fiske, and by multiple regression analyses. The latter analysis was found to demonstrate that SIP scores explained more of the variance in measures of dysfunction (e.g. ADL) than measures of sickness (e.g. self-assessed sickness).

Clinical validity

The SIP places considerable emphasis upon the item categories that make it up, which at the broadest level, correspond to a dimension of physical functioning (Dimension 1: physical categories) versus a dimension of psychosocial functioning (Dimension 2: psychosocial categories). This aspect is seen to allow a demonstration of clinical validity by examining whether clinical conditions load as expected on the internal elements of the SIP.

An example is hyperthyroidism. Bergner et al (1981) hypothesized that for hyperthyroid patients, scores on Dimension 2 (psychosocial categories) would be more highly correlated with thyroid hormone levels than would Dimension 1 scores (physical categories) or overall SIP scores. This was found to be partially supported, in that Dimension 2 scores correlated 0.35 with thyroid hormone levels versus 0.21 for Dimension 1 scores. However, overall SIP levels were more highly correlated again, $r = 0.41$. This was found largely to reflect the action of the independent category 'sleep and rest', which was found to be highly correlated with thyroid level.

While the SIP could not be seen to have passed a test of clinical validity, this test did indicate its potential diagnostic value, i.e. the capacity to pick up what may be unexpected effects of a disease. Temkin et al (1989) have attested to the value of the SIP as a measure of specific disease conditions.

Descriptive validity

Bergner et al (1981) referred to the ability of the SIP to characterize the pattern of dysfunction specific to a given condition. They also stated that it can be difficult or impossible to predict a priori which categories will be most important for a particular sample, and categories should be retained in the instrument even if they make no difference to accounted for variance on the grounds that they contribute to the descriptive capacity of the SIP.

In conclusion

Bergner et al subjected the categories and items of the SIP to considerable analysis to examine the relationships among items, between items and category scores, between items and criterion variables, the frequency of checking of items, and the reliability of items. In this pursuit, a variety of multivariate techniques were used, including stepwise multiple regression, interaction detection analysis, and cluster analysis (resulting in a reduction of the SIP to 12 categories and 136 items).

The SIP illustrates the process whereby the validation of a functional status instrument entails application of a range of convergent and discriminant measures, and the examination of different patient populations. The SIP has been closely examined, and its 'descriptive validity' aspect may have given it considerable value as a diagnostic instrument. On the other hand, it cannot be assumed as valid for all conditions (e.g. with speech pathology), and its method of combining items from different domains into an aggregate SIP score seems to rely upon the assumption that all domains have been sampled comprehensively and equally: content validity seems to have been assumed, not specifically tested.

QUALITY OF WELL-BEING SCALE

The Quality of Well-Being scale (QWB; the term 'Index of Well-Being' or IWB may also be used) was originally developed by Bush and co-workers, and later largely by Kaplan.

Kaplan et al (1989) characterized the QWB as being within the conceptual approach of the SIP and Rand scales; i.e. it focused on

---

Box 9.2   Examples of items from the Quality of Well-Being (QWB) scale

The QWB consists of descriptions of functional states in areas of mobility (3 levels), physical activity (3 levels) and social activity (5 levels), and a list of 21 'symptom/problem complexes'. The test is recommended to be interviewer administered.
   Example of a functional state is:

'Did not drive a car, health-related; did not ride in a car as usual for age (younger than 15 years), health-related, and/or did not use public transportation, health-related; or had or would have used more help than usual for age to use public transportation, health-related.' (Mobility Scale, level 4)

Example of a Symptom Problem Complex is:

'pain, burning, bleeding, itching, or other difficulties with rectum, bowel movements, or urination (passing water).' (CPX no. 8)

(Examples from Kaplan & Anderson 1996)

the impact of disease and disability on function and observable behaviours, such as performance of social role, ability to move around the community, and physical functioning. While developed from a psychometric perspective, Kaplan et al (1989) saw the QWB as providing measures of utility, i.e. the QWB provided a numerical point-in-time expression of well-being that ranges from 0 for death to 1.0 for optimal functioning.

Nature of the Quality of Well-Being scale

The instrument was developed by gathering global assessments of scenarios represented on paper cards, where each card contained an age level (AGE), a functional level (LEV) and a symptom-problem complex (CPX).

There were 4 levels of *age*, e.g. 'older adult (65 years and over)'; while *functional level* was determined by a combination of three characteristics – mobility (5 levels, e.g. drove car and used bus or train without help), physical activity (4 levels, e.g. walked with physical limitations), and social activity (5 levels, e.g. had help with self-care activities). While there were 100 possible function levels (5 × 4 × 5), only 42 of these were considered feasible and ultimately used. There were originally *36 symptom-problem complexes* (CPXs), later grouped to 21, an example of one being 'had pain, burning, bleeding, itching, or other difficulties with rectum, bowel movements, or urination (passing water)'.

Kaplan & Anderson (1988) described the steps involved in building the Health Decision Model as follows.

1. Defining a functional status clarification – first defining a set of mutually exclusive and collectively exhaustive levels of functioning.
2. Classifying symptoms and problems. Kaplan & Anderson (1988) say that in addition to function level clarifications, an exhaustive list of symptoms and problems was generated as 'subjective complaints are an important component of a general health measure because they relate dysfunction to a specific problem', and that 21 CPX complexes represented 'all the possible symptomatic complaints that might inhibit function'.
3. Using preference weights to integrate the three functional subscales and the symptom/problem complexes into a single numerical expression. Human judgement studies were used to

determine weights for the different states, and random samples of citizens from the community were used to evaluate the relative desirability of a good number of health conditions. A mathematical model was developed to describe the consumer decision process, these weights then being used to describe the relative desirability of all the function states on a scale from zero (for death) to 1.0 (for asymptomatic optimum function).

Kaplan et al (1989) further applied the QWB to develop a General Health Policy Model. The aim of the model was to express benefits and side-effects of different health programmes in terms of equivalents of completely well years of life. This entailed the calculation of the expected duration of stay in each QWB level over time, calculating the product and then adding them, to produce what was termed the 'Well Life expectancy', expressed in well years (see e.g. Kaplan & Anderson 1988, Kaplan et al 1989).

According to Kaplan & Anderson (1988) standardized questionnaires are used to clarify individuals into each of the function scale steps, while individuals are classified into the CPX by the one symptom or problem that bothers them most. It is claimed that with structured questions, an interviewer can obtain a classification on the QWB in 11 to 16 minutes.

The QWB has been used to evaluate outcomes in conditions such as AIDS, cystic fibrosis, and arthritis (see Kaplan et al 1989).

Validation

Akin to but seemingly more than the SIP, the QWB appears to rely upon the appropriateness of its initial process of item development and selection. Kaplan et al (1976) explained how an extensive specialty-by-specialty review of medical reference works was conducted to list all the ways diseases and injuries could affect behaviour and role performance. This led to items expressed in terms of behaviours (as opposed to capacities, as such phrasing was reported to cause under-reporting of dysfunction), and embodied in three functional scales, with survey instruments developed to classify a person into one only of the steps of each of the three scales.

The construct validity of the QWB was seen to be established through convergence between its scores and scores of numbers of chronic conditions ($r = -0.96$), number of physician contacts ($r = -0.55$), etc., and discriminant evidence that, e.g. the correlation between QWB on a given day and self-rated well-being on days successively distant decreased systematically (from 0.46 when both relate to the same day, to 0.36 when the well-being measure related to 8 days previously).

A further interesting issue reported by Kaplan et al (1989) was that self-rating of overall health status, where the future as well as the present was taken into account, correlated negligibly with QWB on a given day. That is, QWB (which is specific to a day) gave almost no information about expected future well-being as perceived by individual respondents.

A checking of the Quality of Well-Being model

Balaban et al (1986) re-developed weights for the QWB using a population of sufferers from rheumatoid arthritis. A comparison was made between the QWB score obtained for the 132 scenarios obtained from this population with the scores that would be relevant if Bush's original weights were used. 132 scenarios from combinations of AGE, LEV, and CPX were formed, including 'anchor' scenarios with optimal functioning, and duplicate scenarios to assess respondent consistency.

The task required that subjects were asked to sort each scenario into one of 11 sorting slots, numbered 0 to 10. Zero (0) was marked 'as bad as dying', and 10 as 'completely well'. The data were then analyzed by regressing the global rating given by the subjects against the scenario variables.

Results were analyzed by taking an individual rater's assignment of a score to a particular scenario (category 0–10) and dividing these by 10. The average value given by raters to perfect health scenarios was found to be 0.972. The mean ratings for the 2 pairs of duplicate scenarios were 4.35/4.36, and 5.94/5.93.

The output of the regression analysis gave mobility (MOB) values a range of from 0.000 to 0.147, physical activity (PAC) 0.000 to 0.073, social activity (SAC) 0.000 to 0.126, and CPX 0.000 (no CPX) to 0.654.

In order of potential effect, they were CPX (0.654), MOB (0.147), SAC (0.126), then PAC (0.073). In fact, the smallest CPX (of 21) was 0.130, which was larger than the highest SAC, the highest PAC, and the second highest MOB, which suggests that the CPX tended to swamp the other aspects.

The test for interaction between the variables in the 24 item sub-set was reported to show no significant interactions.

A comparison was made between the QWB score obtained for the 132 scenarios obtained from this population (rheumatoid arthritis sufferers) with the scores that would be relevant if Bush's weights were used, and the two data groups were reported to have a correlation of r = 0.937. However, results for scenarios that compared arthritis-type scenarios only were not given. This leaves open the question as to the accuracy of estimates made by the general public vis a vis patients of specific conditions. It is not surprising that arthritics differed little from the general population when considering non-arthritis conditions, given that both would be equally uninformed.

Problems for the Quality of Well-Being model

Despite Kaplan et al's (1989) efforts to ensure the validity of the QWB (and much effort was invested by Kaplan and co-workers to determine that a rating task could produce interval data, see Ch. 5), the values that emerge from the scale seem quite unexpected.

For example, the highest negative weight associated with PAC is 0.077, which corresponds to 'in wheelchair, did not move or control the movement of wheelchair without help from someone else, or in bed, chair, or couch for most or all of the day (health-related)'. At the same time, CPX-11 'cough, wheezing, or shortness of breath, with or without fever, chills or aching all over' has a weight of −0.257. Because each of the elements of the QWB scale are simply added to 1 (i.e. W = 1 − CPX weight − MOB weight − PAC weight − SAC weight), CPX-11 is estimated to have over 3 *times* the importance of well-being as does the most severe physical activity limitation. This meant that a person totally confined to a wheelchair with no other limitation or symptom would be determined to have a score of 0.923 of total health functioning, while a person with 'cough, wheezing, or shortage of breath' but otherwise totally healthy would have a score of 0.743, which seems almost absurd.

Even quite minor CPX complexes can have a major effect on QWB; for example, wearing eyeglasses (weight = −0.101), having a runny nose (−0.170), and breathing polluted air (−0.101). Such symptom/problem weights were stated by Kaplan & Anderson (1988) to allow the health status index to become 'very sensitive to minor top-end variations in health status'. However, the 'minor' adjustments seem to have the capacity to overwhelm the function scales. Thus the need to wear glasses (-0.101) causes greater reduction in wellness than being in a wheelchair (-0.060 or -0.077). This is not necessarily a problem if other aspects of the function scales always also contribute in such cases, but the fact remains that the scales were deemed to be independent and linearly added in the QWB model.

The QWB may also be criticized on the ground that it was developed on the basis of general community rather than patient or care giver weights. Kaplan & Anderson (1988) defended this aspect by stating that Balaban et al (1986) found weights obtained with arthritis sufferers to be 'remarkably similar to those we obtained from members of the general population' (Kaplan & Anderson 1988, p. 213), while also noting that community weights are general and do not bias policy analysis towards any interest group. Nonetheless, a mix of representative healthcare receivers may have been an alternative way to avoid bias and allowed the QWB to be scaled based on knowledge/experience as opposed to hypothetical estimates.

A further criticism of the QWB is that it did not include measures of social health or mental health. Kaplan responded to this by stating that social support was not an outcome that can serve as a target for healthcare. On the other hand, social functioning was included in the model in the Social Activity Scale. Kaplan saw social function as 'social contacts' (e.g. participation in work, attendance at school), while social support referred to 'social resources' (social life, friendships, family relationships). Kaplan saw the latter as not being in the realm of health policy (asking rhetorically 'would we want to develop a health policy that requires people to have friends?'). However, Hall et al (1989) have shown that the loss of social support as a product of a health state may have a major effect on well-being, and for this reason is worthy of consideration for assessment. Regarding mental health functioning, this was seen to be an intervening variable in affecting physical functioning, and Kaplan claimed, not all that convincingly, that the QWB picked up such effects.

A final question concerns the content validity of the QWB. This was reliant upon the scenarios used to develop the QWB containing accurate representations of the range of possible conditions, or at least a reasonable sub-set. The value of the global ratings elicited by the scenarios was limited by the comprehensiveness/accuracy of scenario descriptions, as well as the knowledge of raters. The gaining of a correlation between arthritis sufferers and the general public on the same scenarios seems more a test of reliability than validity, and it cannot be assumed that content validity has been satisfied.

TORRANCE'S UTILITY MODEL

Torrance (Torrance 1976, 1986, 1987; Torrance et al 1972, 1982) proposed the development of a health utility index for measuring health improvement that was disease and programme independent. An adequate scale was seen to be one that might range from 0 for death (with negative values assigned to fates worse than death) to 1 for good health (defined as the absence of physical, mental, and social disabilities and symptoms). With such an index, every individual could be assigned a score to represent level of health, and the effects of a health programme could be measured in health improvement calculated in health days. The index value assigned to a particular health state was the *utility of that state as perceived by society*, and the model would allocate resources in the health service system so as to maximize their total health utility to society. The health index for the state was intended to represent the utility of that state unaffected by future states that might or might not follow, with prognoses incorporated into the model at a later stage of the analysis.

The techniques proposed to measure the utility of specific health states on a linear scale were the Von Neumann–Morgenstern standard gamble, and a new technique – the 'time tradeoff' method. These were claimed to produce equivalent and reliable results, but with the time tradeoff easier to administer. Further research was advocated to develop a general health utility scale that would eliminate the need to measure specific utilities for each application of the model.

As set out by Torrance (1987), utility referred to the desirability or preference that individuals exhibit for a condition, and a definition of utility was that it is a cardinal measure of the strength of one's preference. The notion as used by Torrance referred to a theory of decision making under uncertainty based on a set of axioms of rational behaviour (Von Neumann & Morgenstern 1953 cited in Torrance 1987). The theory was seen to have face validity in terms of how a problem *should* be approached if a decision is to be made rationally, as defined by the basic axioms of the theory (see Torrance & Feeny 1989), i.e. it is not concerned with modelling how decisions are *actually* carried out.

Testing of instruments

Torrance (1976) noted that a number of health status index models had already been proposed, each defining a set of health states and all requiring a set of numerical weights for these states; these weights were seen to be the weakest aspects of the models. Torrance proposed that a measuring instrument was needed that could reliably and validly quantify preferences for health states, and examined the standard gamble, time tradeoff and category scaling methods.

The subjects used varied with the task, such that only a small university educated group (43 subjects) received all three tasks, the standard gamble being considered too complex for the general public. The university educated group were also re-tested a year later to measure the test re-test reliability of the three techniques. The major subject group was a general public sample (246 subjects), who received the time tradeoff and category rating tasks, as did a small group of patients in a home dialysis programme (29 subjects).

Ten health states were presented, each described by a scenario in narrative form that outlined the physical, emotional and social characteristics of the state.

The standard gamble task consisted of subjects being offered two alternatives, one consisting of an outcome health state with certainty, the other being a gamble with specified probabilities of two possible outcome health states. This task was presented with the assistance of props consisting of a probability wheel and associated colour coded cards.

The time tradeoff task also entailed a choice between two alternatives, but neither was a gamble. Each was a different health state but for differing periods of time.

The category rating task was a complex one, requiring simultaneous assessments of the effects of both the illness state per se, and the affect of being in that state for varying periods of time until death. The task entailed presenting subjects with a 100 millimetre line marked 'Death, least desirable' at one end and 'Healthy, most desirable' at the other, and they were told that it represented 101 equal interval categories. For each health state scenario presented, subjects were asked to mark three lines on the 'desirability line', one corresponding to the relative desirability of being in that state for 3 months then death, one for being in that state for 8 years then death, and a final line indicating the relative desirability of being in that state for the remainder of their normal life expectancy.

The results were that subjects found the time tradeoff task the easiest, the standard gamble slightly more difficult (but probably impossible without the props), and the direct scaling task the most difficult. Only the time tradeoff task was considered to be capable of being executed without a well-trained interviewer.

Measures of internal consistency (coefficient of reliability) provided correlations of 0.77 and 0.79 for the standard gamble and time tradeoff correspondingly, with standard errors of estimate of 0.125 and 0.135 correspondingly, and test re-test reliabilities of 0.53 and 0.62 correspondingly. The category scaling task test re-test reliability was found to be 0.49.

Approach to validity

The validity of the tasks was assessed on the assumption that the standard gamble was a criterion measure as it was valid by definition and it was not necessary or appropriate to validate the measures obtained from this task.

The other two tasks were compared to the standard gamble, obtaining uncorrected correlations of 0.65 and 0.36 for the time tradeoff and category rating tasks correspondingly. In essence, it was concluded that the time tradeoff was the method of choice, being simpler to apply, of relatively high validity, and if anything, more reliable. The category rating task was condemned as the poorest technique, its only redeeming virtue being its potential lower cost.

Sackett & Torrance (1978) reported further analysis of the general population interviews using the time tradeoff task, looking at variables that affected utility estimates within the group. They found effects of:

* Age – older subjects provided lower utility scores for dialysis and transplantation, and higher scores for hospital confinement for an unnamed infectious disease.
* Socio-economic class – hospital confinement tended to have higher utility for those living in lower income neighbourhoods.

- Duration of illness state – the mean daily utility was less for lengthy illness states than short duration ones.
- Label given to the illness state – e.g. use of the label 'tuberculosis' gave higher health state utilities than 'unnamed contagious disease'.
- Experience with the condition – home dialysis patients gave a higher utility to home dialysis than did the general public.

It should be clear that Torrance (e.g. Feeny & Torrance 1989, Torrance & Feeny 1989) saw the standard gamble as being basically different to, say, the rating scale approach.

The standard gamble was seen to provide numerical values that may be termed utilities, while the rating scale provided numbers more properly termed values; the reason being that the standard gamble values health states under uncertainty while the rating scale values health states under certainty. Only the standard gamble was seen to directly measure Von Neumann–Morgenstern utilities, all other instruments were at best approximations. As noted by Mulley (1989), the measurement technique was seen to be validated based on axioms of rational choice.

This approach does not seem to allow for the limitations of human cognitive ability. It assumes, e.g. that probabilities and values for states can be manipulated according to the axioms of the model. To the extent to which, say, the standard gamble task is not computed as expected by the model, then the parameters derived from an analysis using such a task are likely to be in error. The value placed on a given health state cannot necessarily be derived from a decomposition of the results from a complex decision under uncertainty. The approach is quite different to that used by those concerned with measuring a psychological construct. If QoL is interpreted as psychological well-being, then the aim is to develop a tool which can provide consistent and valid estimates of well-being depending upon health state, not normatively modelling a decision process.

Development of a multi-attribute utility scale

Torrance (Torrance et al 1982, Boyle et al 1983) reported the application of multi-attribute utility (MAU) theory to measure social preferences for health states. It should be noted that multi-attribute utility theory was not seen to introduce any new methods of measuring preference, but rather introduced a way of selecting specific preferences to be measured and combining them into a mathematical model of the subject's utility structure (Torrance 1986).

Torrance et al (1982) described a measure of health status that categorized states using four attributes. These were mobility and physical activity (6 levels), self care and role activity (5 levels), emotional well-being and social activity (4 levels), and health problem (8 levels). Each individual was to be classified using 1 level only for each of the four attributes. The standard gamble task was not used for the purpose of developing the MAU, due to its complexity and difficulty of administration. Instead, a simple category rating task was used to make single attribute measurements, with respondents asked to rate the desirability or undesirability of a health state relative to other health states and relative to the reference states 'health' and 'dead'. Time tradeoff was also used to make multi-attribute measurements. The relative value that members of society attach to the various possible health states was determined through measuring aggregated social preference (utility) for each of the possible 960 states in the classification system using a random sample of parents of school-aged children from the general population.

This general approach was described by Torrance (1986, see also Torrance 1987) as representing the idea of a multi-attribute health state classification system, based on the concept that health state can be defined in terms of a number of attributes (the QWB system of Bush/Kaplan is given as another example of this).

Regarding who should provide utility values, Torrance seemed quite flexible. He suggested that informed members of the public are the appropriate subjects for gathering utilities regarding public policy decisions, although he noted that obtaining informed subjects, in the sense that the subject truly understands what the health state is like, is a very difficult issue. He also stated that the simplest way of obtaining utility values was to use judgement to estimate it, either by the analyst or by a few physicians or other experts (however, the literature or other forms of measurement was advocated if the analysis showed the results were sensitive to utility values). Torrance also considered that in some applications the relevant health states for which utilities are required are simply the health states of the patients in the study, and there the patients are available to give those utilities – this is seen to avoid the need to prepare a description of the health state for use by subjects.

Torrance's approach to validity appeared to change progressively. Torrance (1986) noted that an alternative approach to validity (other than assuming the necessary validity of the standard gamble) is that health state utilities measure the overall QoL associated with the health state, and a test of validity is to determine if the utility measure is correlated significantly with other trusted measures of HQoL.

Torrance's early MAU scale underwent little validation that would be accepted by those with a background in psychological measurement.

SF-36 (MEDICAL OUTCOMES STUDY 36 ITEM SHORT-FORM HEALTH SURVEY)

First reported in the literature by Ware & Sherbourne (1992), the SF-36 has become probably the most widely used of all health status measures. It was described as reflecting the increasing consensus regarding the patient's point of view in monitoring medical care outcomes, and the need for a standardized heath status survey that was comprehensive, psychometrically sound, and brief. See also McHorney et al (1993) and Ware (1993).

Box 9.3 Examples of items from the MOS 36-item short-form health survey (SF-36)

The SF-36 consists of a 36 item questionnaire suitable for self-completion. Scores are provided corresponding to eight sub-scales: physical functioning; role-physical; bodily pain; social functioning; mental health; role-emotional; vitality, and general health perceptions.
   Examples of items are:

Item 1   *In general, would you say your health is:*
         Excellent ☐   *Very good* ☐   *Good* ☐   *Fair* ☐   *Poor* ☐

Item 5   *During the past 4 weeks have you had any of the following problems with your work or other regular daily activities as a result of any emotional problems (such as feeling depressed or anxious)?*

         *a) Cut down on the **amount of time** you spent on work or other*
             activities (yes/no)
         *b) **Accomplished less** than you would like (yes/no)*
         *c) Didn't do work or other activities as **carefully** as usual (yes/no)*

(Examples from Wilkin et al 1993)

The SF-36 offered a 36-item questionnaire forming a multi-item scale measuring health concepts described as most frequently represented in widely-used health surveys. These were: physical functioning; role limitations because of physical health problems; bodily pain; social functioning; general mental health (psychological distress and psychological well-being), role limitations because of emotional problems; vitality (energy/fatigue), and general health perceptions. Most of the items were reported to have been adapted from instruments in use for 20–40 years or longer.

It was stated from the outset that while the SF-36 included eight distinct health status concepts and one item measuring self-reported health transition, important health concepts were not represented. Among the omitted were seen to be: health distress, family functioning, sexual functioning, cognitive functioning, and sleep disorders. It was also noted that for studies of severely ill populations, it may be desirable to add a supplementary battery of items to represent the extreme low end of the continuum (the example was given of the physical functioning scale, which includes only one item focusing on daily self-care activities).

McHorney et al (1993) discussed the validity of the SF-36, described as the 'interpretability and meaningfulness of scores'. The instrument was subjected to construct validation, seen to entail:

- specifying the domain of variables, i.e. preparing a blue print of constructs
- establishing the internal structure of observed variables
- verifying theoretical relationships between scale scores and external criteria.

Both in construction and evaluation, the development of the SF-36 followed a traditional psychometric approach, using factor analysis to identify constructs hypothesized to underlie broad physical and mental dimensions, and then factors underlying the sub-scales.

The data came from the Medical Outcomes Study, which gathered data in Boston, Chicago and Los Angeles on over 2000 patients, who were given both clinical examinations and extensive questionnaires, therefore allowing patients to be allocated to different medical groups (e.g. minor chronic medical, chronic medical, psychiatric only, both medical and psychiatric).

The pattern of correlations between sub-scales and two extracted dimensions of physical and mental were examined, and it was concluded that patterns of high correlation (e.g. mental health sub-scale with the mental dimension – congruent validity), and low correlation (e.g. role physical with mental dimension – discriminant validity) were as expected.

Moreover, the pattern of sub-scale scores differed as expected according to the clinical status of the patients involved, e.g. patients classified as minor medical had higher 'role physical' sub-scale scores (representing less deficits) than patients classified as serious medical. The data also allowed scale calibration, e.g. it was concluded that a difference of 27 points in the mental health scale reflected the impact of serious depressive symptoms.

The primary notion of validation used by the SF-36 was that the pattern of scores was as expected. Criterion-related validation was not attempted. While it is frequently maintained that criterion-related validation is not possible (Aaronson et al 2002), this position seems more a convention than obvious. As argued earlier in this book (see Ch. 5 under 'Patient Global Self-ratings' and 'Global Ratings as Criterion Measures in Test Development'), once one applies an instrument to a specific patient population, global patient report of HQoL is available to provide at least a proxy-criterion measure.

Ware & Sherbourne (1992) noted that the popularity of the SF-36 appeared to be largely driven by its brevity and comprehensiveness, achieved by using very short multi-item scales, with the potential for 'an unacceptable loss of measurement precision'. It was seen to be supported based on analyses of group-level data, but that the appropriateness of the instrument for monitoring outcomes for individual patients was unclear.

The SF-36 has gone on to be probably the most widely used HQoL measure of all time, applied to a very broad range of illness conditions, producing thousands of reports, and issues of prominent journals dedicated to SF-36 related research (e.g. *The Journal of Clinical Epidemiology* 51(11), 1998).

The SF-36 has also experienced ongoing development, although not without criticism. For discussion regarding the addition of Physical Component Summary (PCS) and Mental Component Summary (MCS) summary measures, see Taft et al (2001a, b) and Ware & Kosinski (2001).

There are periodic reports of shortcomings, e.g. Littlewood et al (2001) reported it to be insensitive to changing haemoglobin levels in patients undergoing chemotherapy (unlike the cancer-specific instruments that were also used); Wolinsky et al (1998) judged the SF-36 to be inferior to a modified version of the Chronic Heart Failure Questionnaire (CHQ) for use among outpatients known to have coronary artery disease and/or congestive heart failure; Nortvedt et al (2000) found the SF-36 to be less able to detect the effects of disease progression in multiple sclerosis patients than the RAND-36 health status survey (the RAND-36 has identical items but is scored differently, see Hays et al (1998) and Hays & Morales (2001)).

In conclusion, as with any instrument, the SF-36 is liable to be insensitive and/or misleading when used for the wrong purpose.

SUMMARY AND CONCLUSIONS

Sickness impact profile

The development of the SIP entailed gathering a very large number of descriptions of behaviour associated with different health states. Judges were later used to scale all items individually from minimally to severely dysfunctional, and items showing excessive inter-judge variation were deleted. The ability of different scoring methods to predict global assessments of SIP profiles was then examined and an extensive examination followed, of the correspondence between SIP scores and other measures, across a range of different patient populations.

A major strength of the development process of the SIP was its pursuit of 'descriptive validity' – the capacity to characterize a very broad range of illness effects; the willingness to closely examine and report the SIP's shortcomings (e.g. with speech pathology patients) was another.

In many ways, the development of the SIP was admirable (if resulting in a somewhat cumbersome instrument), although like all instruments it too had its flaws: the use of judges with limited experience of illness behaviours to weight items seems to have been one.

Quality of Well-Being scale

Regarding the QWB scale, despite Kaplan et al's efforts to ensure its validity, the values of the QWB seem quite unexpected. Moreover, its failure to assess social effects of illness (e.g. loss of social support) or mental health functioning may be seen as indicating overly limited content. A further difficulty is its reliance on general community rather than patient or care giver weights (an aspect recognized as more questionable since the demonstration that people change their minds about illness states once they enter them; cf. Loewenstein & Schkade 1997).

Torrance's utility model

Torrance's MAU theory to measure social preferences for health states, used a random sample of parents of school-aged children from the general population. Torrance argued that informed members of the public are the appropriate subjects for gathering utilities regarding public policy decisions, but also noted that in some applications, the relevant health states for which utilities are required are simply the health states of the patients in the study and the patients could provide those utilities. Torrance's early MAU scale underwent little validation that would be accepted by those with a background in psychological measurement.

SF-36

In contrast to the QWB and Torrance's MAU measure, the SF-36 was developed based on the notion that the patient's point of view in monitoring medical care outcomes is of key importance. Considerable effort was invested in construct validation, including specifying the domain of variables and verifying theoretical relationships between scale scores and external criteria. Both in construction and evaluation, the development of the SF-36 followed a traditional psychometric approach.

There was also explicit recognition of the SF-36's shortcomings. Ware & Sherbourne (1992) noted that the popularity of the SF-36 appeared to be largely driven by its brevity and comprehensiveness, achieved by using very short multi-item scales, with the potential for 'an unacceptable loss of measurement precision'. It was also stated at the outset that the SF-36 omitted important health concepts (e.g. health distress, family functioning, sexual functioning, cognitive functioning, sleep disorders), and that floor effects might be a problem if severely ill populations were assessed.

Since then, the SF-36 has gone on to be probably the most widely used HQoL measure of all time. However, it should always be borne in mind that the SF-36 is capable of being insensitive and/or misleading if used for an inappropriate population or purpose.

KEY POINTS

- There is considerable variation in the ways that tests are developed, resulting in distinct differences in capacity and final form. As a result all tests tends to have unique strengths and weaknesses.
- As stated often in this book, it is essential that each test is examined carefully to ensure it is appropriate for the intended purpose, with its weaknesses recognized and where possible compensated for.

For further brief reviews of health outcome measures, see Wilkin et al (1993), McDowell & Newell (1996), and Bowling (1997).

10

Evaluating an instrument

AIMS OF CHAPTER

- To encourage the evaluation of instruments

- To provide an intuitive short-hand method for test evaluation

- To provide a template for a more extensive assessment

EXAMINE INSTRUMENTS CAREFULLY

Instruments tend to be developed then promoted. As candidly observed by Hyland, 'The last person you should come to for a recommendation about QoL scales is someone who is an author (of one) – including myself' (Hyland 2002, p. 599).

With some exceptions (e.g. Bergner's rigorous and uncompromising assessment of the Sickness Impact Profile [SIP]: see Ch. 9), instruments that succeed in reaching a wide audience can become resistant to improvement. Both the author(s) and the audience may wish to affirm the merit of the instrument. The desire for a standard instrument discourages the reporting of failure, and hinders change leading to improvement (see also Epstein & Lydick 1995).

In addition there can be little appreciation that tests are not valid, uses are (see Ch. 4). As a result, those seeking a test may accept that a test has been 'validated' solely because it has been cited often. A circularity may operate:

citation   →   adoption

   ↑   ↓

adoption   ←   citation

It is important that the validity of tests is determined by means other than 'valid by authority' or 'valid by citation'. This requires an understanding of the nature of tests, and the rationale of the statistical evidence (e.g. Cronbach's Alpha).

To repeat, the most important notion to understand is that tests may be appropriate in one setting but not in another. Tests are not valid per se.

SHORT-HAND ASSESSMENT

Instruments are frequently not well documented, and there can be insufficient evidence to comprehensively assess even commonly used instruments. A useful short-hand approach is to consider two main types of evidence that bear on the validity of tests. These are:

- the adequacy of the process of construction
- correspondence between the test's scores and direct measures of the construct.

The adequacy of the process of construction

The basic point is that to evaluate a test, one needs to go through the same steps as would be needed to construct it in the first place. Was the instrument constructed in such a way that one would 'prima facie' expect it to accurately measure what it is proposed to measure? Was validity built into a test from the outset? This entails the following questions:

Were the purpose of the test and the concept (construct)
to be measured clearly defined?

Was there clear specification of the purpose of the instrument? Was the construct (the property that is to be estimated) clearly stated? Was an operational definition of the construct clearly stated?

Was an adequate range of content areas assessed?

When measuring health-related quality of life (HQoL)/health status, the most important domains of content (e.g. mobility, pain, etc.) will depend upon the patient's illness. The sampling of these dimensions is central to validity. For example, for cystic fibrosis patients, stamina and breathing difficulty are among the greatest concerns, and should be considered for inclusion during the process of instrument formation.

Shumaker et al (1997) described key questions in assessing HQoL measures as whether the necessary dimensions were included or not, and whether or not these dimensions were assessed with sufficient breadth, depth, validity, reliability and responsiveness to change. They noted general factors for HQoL as including social, physical and cognitive functioning, mobility and self care, and emotional well-being.

Were clear and unambiguous items prepared to represent each domain and were analyses conducted to select the most valid items?

Careful item preparation to represent each domain, followed by analyses to select the most valid items, is essential. An item needs to be shown to belong in a scale based on both the construct definition and the results of item analyses.

If a global score was provided, were sub-scales/domains combined/weighted in such a way as to ensure the global score was valid?

The number properties of the scale and sub-scales need to be tested, and sub-scales/domains weighted (and/or a scoring algorithm developed), such that the magnitude of the global score can be expected to be a good estimate of the construct being estimated.

Was there evidence of correspondence between test scores and direct measures?

The ultimate means of determining if an instrument is adequately assessing HQoL/health status, is its ability to predict (or otherwise correspond to) evidence of the patients well-being/functional status. There is rarely a reason why this should not include attempts to gather patient or 'expert' report of this. Anastasi (1990) noted that, fundamentally, all procedures for determining test validity are concerned with the relationships between performance on the test and other independently observable facts about the behaviour characteristics under consideration.

A TEMPLATE FOR EVALUATING A TEST

This template provides a general structure and content, and specific headings and sub-headings, for reporting the evaluation of a test. It represents the author's views, but has been influenced by content drawn from 'A Suggested Outline for Test Evaluation' in Anastasi (1990), the instrument review criteria proposed by the Medical Outcomes Trust (Aaronson et al 2002), and the suggestions of Shumaker et al (1997).

It needs to be clear that the following represents a brief overview only. Virtually all of the information in this book is relevant to test evaluation.

Specification of intended use of test by the evaluator

The following concerns *the requirements of the test user*. By stating these formally, a comparison can be readily made with candidate instruments.

Purpose

What is the purpose of the test? This includes the decision(s) to be guided.

The construct

What is the construct that the test is to assess? For example, is it subjective well-being, functional status, self-perceived health, etc?

The population

Who is the test to be applied to? This includes sub-populations (e.g. age range, ethnic groups, illnesses/disabilities, etc.)

Source of information

Who is to provide the information required to complete the test? Is the test to be patient based, clinician based, care giver based, etc.

Presentation mode

How is the test to be administered? Is it self-administered via a booklet, interviewer-administered, computer based, etc.

Content

What is the type of content required? What are the dimensions to be assessed, etc.

Criteria

What are the criteria the instrument needs to meet? This includes:

- Practical needs, e.g. length, resources required to administer the test
- Output, e.g. areas of importance to patient, sub-scale scores for each area, overall score
- Ability to guide clinical decisions
- Other characteristics, covered as extensively as possible.

The remainder of the template concerns the candidate test instrument.

Overview of the candidate test

- Title, author, publisher, publication date and manuals date, cost
- Intended purpose (by developer), and intended population (by developer)
- Conceptual basis of the test, if apparent (classical sum scale, Rasch, Item Response Theory (IRT), etc.)
- Presentation mode intended by developer (self-administered [booklet], interviewer scored, computer based, etc.)
- Number by type of items (Likert, Guttman, visual analogue scale (VAS), etc.)
- Structure (sub-tests with separate scores plus aggregate score, etc.).

Note that the properties of an instrument are context specific. An instrument that works well for one purpose or in one setting or population may not do so when applied for another purpose or in another setting or population.

Adequacy of the test construction method

The following need to be taken into account in assessing the adequacy of the test construction method.

Method of development

Tests may be based on Classical Test Theory (CTT) summed scales, Guttman, Rasch/IRT, etc. or a mixture of scale types. Given the scale form(s), the adequacy of the processes followed should be considered.

Content

The methods for developing the content of the instrument, including both the nature of the items and the processes used to select and refine the items should be considered. These include:

- Method of identifying necessary content (literature, healthcare personnel, patients)
- Method of forming and testing instructions and items
- Revision and pre-testing of items and instructions.

Scaling of items, grouping of items to form the scale or sub-scales, the scoring of the scales, and interval properties of scores

The following should be considered:

- The conceptual and empirical basis for the scores of items that have been allocated distinguishing values (e.g. for Guttman or Thurstonian scales).
- If a single unidimensional scale, the conceptual and empirical basis for identifying which items will be grouped together to form a single scale, and the procedure and rationalization for deriving scale scores from raw scores.
- If a summed scale, items should be inter-correlated as indicated by item-total correlations (CTT model). Information from factor analysis may be available.

- Items of tests based on the Rasch Model/IRT should be spread along a continuum in an ordered manner as expected given their individual nature, fit statistics should have been examined to demonstrate adequacy of the model, unidimensionality should have been explored, etc.

Combination/weighting of sub-tests to score the overall test

If multiple unidimensional sub-scales have been combined to provide a global score, a clear rationale for the combination method should be apparent.

Procedures for developing the meaningfulness of the test

Steps taken to aid interpretation of the scores should be considered.

Evaluating the completed test

Practical evaluation

The following should be considered:

- Clarity of directions
- Tester qualifications and/or training required, and the availability of the training
- Ease of administration, ease of conducting, and ease of scoring
- Face validity to testers and testees
- Respondent burden, i.e. the ease of completion by the test-takers.

Appropriateness of content

There should be an assessment of whether or not the content of the instrument seems appropriate given its intended use, based on the literature, professional opinion, and patient report; this should cover:

- Inclusion of relevant domains
- Adequate coverage of (each) domain in terms of range, depth of items
- Clarity of items.

Reliability issues

Test reliability is the degree to which an instrument is free from random error. Reliability places a limit on the degree to which the test can measure what it is intended to.

Reliability is encouraged by homogeneity of content within multi-item tests (i.e. high correlations among test items), the most common approach for assessing internal consistency being Cronbach's Alpha. A second aspect of reliability is reproducibility, i.e. stability of an instrument over time (test-retest), and inter-rater agreement.

Ideally both internal consistency and reproducibility should be assessed, with reliability estimates or standard errors reported for both total score and sub-scale scores (where applicable). Reliability estimates or standard errors of measurement should be presented for the various population with which the instrument is to be used (disease populations, language or cultural groups, etc.). There should be a description of the method employed to collect reliability data, including characteristics of the sample and the testing conditions.

Evidence that the test can measure what it is required to measure

Validity refers to the degree to which a scale measures what *the user* desires it to measure. Validity is related to the application of an instrument, not to the instrument itself, and is a matter of degree. The primary assessments that may be made are:

Predicting a criterion, e.g. patient global report (criterion-related validity). Criterion-related validation procedures indicate the effectiveness of a test in predicting an individual's specified performance or report, i.e. it considers evidence that scores of the instrument are appropriately related to a criterion measure. When data related to criterion validity are presented, a clear rationale for the choice of the criterion measure is essential.

Demonstrating differences between groups. The test should be assessed to see if individuals or populations hypothesized to differ (on the construct being assessed) do so. If expected differences are found, the test is supported. If not, there may be a fault in the theory underlying the construct, the measure of the construct, or the treatment/distinction assumed to provide the difference.

**Longitudinal sensitivity or 'responsiveness': detecting changes
due to treatment.**   A HQoL measure needs to be able to discriminate between levels of a disease condition due to disease course
or treatment. 'Responsiveness' refers to ability to detect change.
Assessing responsiveness requires asking whether the test can
detect differences in outcomes that are important, even if those
differences are small.

Common methods of evaluating responsiveness include
comparing scale scores before and after an intervention that is
expected to affect the construct, and comparing changes in scale
scores with changes in other related measures that are assumed to
move in the same direction as the target measure. In this latter category, care needs to be taken that the other measure is appropriate: it is desirable to avoid using another test.

The measure needs to be able to detect a worsening state in
patients who already have a relatively poor QoL, and an improvement for patients whose QoL is relatively good (i.e. not display
floor and ceiling effects).

Ability to signal adaptation

For some purposes, it may be desirable that the test indicates
whether a change in the patient's condition has occurred but is
being concealed by some form of adaptation. The inclusion of
multiple measures of the construct may assist this. Patient report
that may be adaptation-sensitive, such as global report of life satisfaction, HQoL, or affect, may be supplemented by HQoL predictions derived from test content that is based on observables.
Alternatively, carer-based or other indirect and/or objective variables may be available.

Interpretation of scores

Is the score interpretable and can judgements be made regarding
the clinical significance of the score (Shumaker et al 1997)?

Interpretability is the degree to which one can assign qualitative
meaning to an instrument's quantitative scores. Interpretability of
a measure is facilitated by information that translates a quantitative score or change in scores to a qualitative category that has clinical or commonly understood meaning.

There are various types of information that can aid in the interpretation of scores:

- comparative data on the distribution of scores derived from a variety of defined population groups, including when relevant and possible, a representative sample of the general population
- information on the relationship of scores to clinically recognized conditions or need for specific treatments
- changes in scores to commonly-recognized life events (such as the impact of losing a job)
- relevant events (such as death or need for institutional care).

Training required in the test

Where tests require the training of test administrators, it needs to be checked that the training is available, affordable, and is unlikely to be a significant source of test score variation.

Application to diverse groups

Where the population to be assessed is culturally diverse, some sub-groups may be poorly served by the test. This issue needs to be considered in its own right, as well as part of 'reliability', 'validity', etc. Basically, does the measure provide equally valid results across different age, cultural and sub-cultural groups? Instruments that were developed in Anglo-Celtic middle class populations may not perform satisfactorily with low income and/or ethnically diverse groups.

Questions to be asked include:

- are the key HQoL issues comparable across the groups to which the test will be applied?
- has this been systematically addressed in the development and assessment of the measure, i.e. has the measure been developed to serve a range of populations?

Summary evaluation of the test

The major strengths and weaknesses of the test are outlined, cutting across all areas, and including any shortcomings that may be suspected but not confirmed.

The likely ability of the test to meet the requirements of its intended use (as set out in 'Specification of Intended Use of Test by the Evaluator' earlier) is discussed and stated.

SUMMARY

There can be a tendency to assume that the test must be okay, or to say 'who am I to say that it is not?' Any such disposition should play no part in selecting a test. This chapter aimed to provide a road map for examining tests.

> ### KEY POINTS IN SELECTING A TEST
>
> - Tests need to be evaluated for the purpose that is required of them. Tests are not valid per se. A test may be excellent for one purpose, but fail completely for another.
> - Multi-item/multi-domain instruments have the ability to lay out the dimensions of relevance, so possessing diagnostic value as well as potential for greater reliability and validity. Yet single-item patient estimates of global HQoL have a role too, both in situations where a multi-domain or even multi-item measure is not essential (a simple, clearly defined and focused visual analogue scale is better than a complex instrument that is not measuring what is intended), and as a check on a more comprehensive instrument.
> - Sometimes the best solution is three measures: a specific measure to target the condition, a generic measure to detect unintended consequences of treatment, and a single item to gather a global report from the patient.

> ### QUOTABLE QUOTE
>
> *Competent test users understand and appreciate the limitations of the tests they use, as well as how those limitations might be compensated for by data from other sources.*
>
> (Cohen & Swerdlick 1999, p. 14)

See Awad et al (1997), Shumaker et al (1997), Sen et al (1999), Bonsignore et al (2001), Aaronson et al (2002), for further views relating to assessing instruments.

11

Topics of special interest

AIMS OF CHAPTER

To consider topics that are of considerable importance and that are
in transition, namely:

- Interpreting quality of life scores for individual patients

- Cross-cultural application issues

- Measuring 'utilities'

- The problem of missing or incomplete data

- Dynamic measures: measuring health-related behaviour to
  prevent future outcomes

There are a number of issues critical to the most effective application of patient-centred health outcome measures that are unresolved or in transition. This chapter considers some of them.

INTERPRETING QUALITY OF LIFE SCORES FOR INDIVIDUAL PATIENTS

So far there has been relatively little uptake in clinical practice of health-related quality of life (HQoL) measures for the assessment of individual patients (Liang 2000). This is likely to be in part due to lack of experience with such measures. Clinicians are familiar with changes in physiological measures that indicate an altered treatment plan due to their training and experience, but HQoL measures have been primarily research tools and are not part of the experience of most clinicians (Jaeschke et al 1989, Wyrwich & Wolinsky 2000). There have also been few studies of the way in which HQoL measures relate to clinically important changes (Liang 2000).

This issue is now recognized, with a spate of papers addressing the issue of how to interpret HQoL scores for clinical purposes (e.g. Erickson 2000, Guyatt 2000, Kaplan et al 2000, Testa 2000, Norman et al 2001, Samsa 2001, Cella et al 2002a, Hajiro & Nishimura 2002, Jones 2002).

The thrust has been to identify the minimal clinical importance difference (MCID or MID) for an instrument, 'the smallest difference in score in the domain of interest which patients perceive as beneficial and which would mandate, in the absence of troublesome side effects and excessive cost, a change in the patient's (healthcare) management' (Jaeschke et al 1989).

The statistical analysis of clinical trials using HQoL measures is usually not a problem, as the interpretation of trial effects may be based on detecting statistically significant changes in mean HQoL differences. Such effects are inherently related to sample size. The magnitude of a statistically significant HQoL change for a group may have no relation to a meaningful HQoL difference for individual patients (Norman et al 2001, Wyrwich & Wolinsky 2000, Sloan et al 2002b).

Anchor-based methods for establishing linkage between health-related quality of life scores and clinical events

Anchor-based methods examine the relationship between scores on the instrument whose interpretation is under question 'the target instrument' and some independent measure 'an anchor' (Guyatt et al 2002). The following description of anchor-based methods follows the typology of Jones (2002).

Patient-based anchors

The most common way of identifying what constitutes a MCID has been to link the change in scores on individual instruments to patients' global judgements on outcome. Norman et al (2001) give the example of patients being asked if they had 'got better, stayed about the same, or got worse'. If they reported having improved or worsened, they rated the degree of change from 1 to 7. The MID is then taken as the mean change on the HQoL scale of the patients who score 1 to 3.

Because health status questionnaires treat each patient as if they were a 'typical' patient (questionnaire items forming a lowest common denominator of similarity between patients), it is reasonable to use threshold scores that are also standard for that population. However, Jones (2002) points out that patients will differ in the value they place upon disturbances in different domains, and so there will, in fact, be inter-individual differences in the threshold score for clinical significance.

The use of patient ratings to obtain MCIDs has been criticized by Norman et al (1997), who argued that patients global change estimates were affected by factors such as incorrect estimates of prior state, and uncertain reliability. Wyrwich & Wolinsky (2000) proposed a clinical interpretation of an individual's HQoL change by the patient's own doctor in consultation with the patient, arguing that clinical assessments of change in health status and their treatment implications must be included if meaningful intra-individual HQoL change standards are to be developed.

Clinician-based anchors

Jaeschke et al (1989) reported establishing a minimum clinically important difference (for the CRQ) via discussion among a group of clinicians who had administered the questionnaire to patients in three clinical studies. A consensus was reached that most patients with an increase of three points on the dyspnoea domain had experienced a reduction in dyspnoea that was important to them in their daily lives.

This approach has not generally been pursued. As noted by Wyrwich & Wolinsky (2000), there is evidence that doctors often underestimate or fail to recognize limitations and symptoms that patients report (e.g. see Ch. 1 under 'The Recognition That Patients Have a Distinctive View of Their Health'), and when doctors are asked to estimate global HQoL change scores they often consult their patients – thus patients are the most direct and error-free source of data.

External criterion anchors

HQoL scores may also be compared to an external criterion. Jones (2002) referred to 'criterion referencing' using the occurrence of hospital admission or death. Thus Osman et al (1997) obtained scores on the St George's Respiratory Questionnaire (SGRQ) from patients discharged from hospital following an acute exacerbation of chronic obstructive pulmonary disease (COPD). They tracked patients who had been re-admitted to hospital or died, versus those who had had neither major event. The difference in test score between these two groups (at baseline) was identified (4.8 units, 95% CI 1.6 and 8.0 units).

Lydick & Epstein (1996) suggested that it is helpful to anchor HQoL results to clinical and other outcomes, such as a 3-point change on the Chronic heart Failure Questionnaire indicating effect of digoxin, or a 10-point change in Brief Psychiatric Rating Scale indicating a likely psychotic exacerbation within 3 weeks. Many such anchors have been explored by Ware et al (e.g. see Ware & Keller 1996).

Methods of interpreting anchor-based changes in health status measurements

The proportion who benefit. Once a MCID (or MID) has been determined, the mean treatment effect may be compared with the MCID: if the effect is less than the MCID, it is judged to be sub-clinical.

In making this comparison, Norman et al (2001) suggested using the lower confidence interval of the MCID (although a problem is that the size of the confidence interval depends on the number of observations used to make the estimate): the proportion benefiting from a treatment can then be determined by counting the number of patients in the treatment group above the MCID versus the number in the control group above the MCID.

NNT: number of patients need to treat (for one to exceed MCID).
Some patients within a population may have a worthwhile benefit from treatment even though the mean effect for the population
may be less than the MCID.

Norman et al (2001) describe how once patients have been categorized into those in whom the MCID was exceeded and those
in whom it did not (i.e. the proportion who benefit), the difference
in proportions can be converted to the number of patients who
would need to be treated to prevent one event (NNT).

Use of scenarios. Jones (2002) gave examples of converting the
SGRQ thresholds into scenarios (brief descriptions of patient states)
to provide further meaning for clinicians of a, say, 4 unit change in
the questionnaire.

Distribution-based methods

Distribution-based methods rely on expressing an effect in terms
of the underlying distribution of results. Effects may be expressed
in terms of standard deviation units (SDs) as the Effect Size (ES).
Measures are then dependent on the distribution of change scores
(see e.g. Guyatt et al 2002, Norman et al 2001), i.e. interpretation is
not straight forward as effect sizes are affected by the homogeneity of the sample used to calculate them.

Guyatt et al (2002) point out that distribution-based methods
differ from anchor-based methods in that they interpret results in
terms of the relation between the magnitude of effect and measures
of variability in results. However, the values are easy to generate
compared to generating an anchor-based interpretation.

Unfortunately, SDs have little intuitive meaning to clinicians.
Guyatt et al (2002) suggested that clinicians would gain experience
with SDs and might be educated with standards such as changes
of 0.2 SDs representing small changes, of 0.5 SDs moderate changes,
and 0.8 SDs large changes (Cohen 1988, cited in Guyatt et al 2002).
These SDs are based on group means; others have suggested larger
change requirements (see Wyrwich & Wolinsky 2000).

An alternative is the Standard Error of Measurement (SEM),
which has the virtue of being sample independent (Anastasi &
Urbina 1997, Nunnally & Bernstein 1994). A one or two SEM
change has been suggested as a grounds for considering that
meaningful individual change has occurred (see Wyrwich &
Wolinsky 2000).

Bridging the two methods

Norman et al (2001) argued that there must be an association between distribution and anchor-based approaches methods given that larger effect sizes mean that a greater proportion of the treatment group will fall above any chosen MCID than the control group (although noting that the two approaches could conceivably lead to opposite conclusions, e.g. where the effect size was large but not the MCID). To investigate this they investigated the relationship between ES expressed in SDs, and the proportion of patients benefiting from treatment (pB). This was conducted using simulation based on the normal distribution for various values of the ES and the MCID, and then assessed agreement of the simulation with data from studies of asthma and respiratory disease.

Norman et al reported that the simulation showed a near linear relationship between ES and pB, and a high level of agreement with the empirical data. It was concluded that the proportion of patients who will benefit from treatment can be directly estimated from the ES (and is nearly independent of the choice of MID), in other words, ES and anchor-based approaches provided equivalent information. See also Samsa (2001).

Wyrwich et al (2002) also found a close correspondence between one MCID (anchor-based approach) and a criterion of 1 SEM with the Chronic Heart Failure Questionnaire (CHQ) and Chronic Respiratory Disease Questionnaire (CRQ) measures. Others have advocated higher SEM values (see Guyatt et al 2002).

Overall, the evidence is that distribution-based methods are simpler and may prove extremely useful.

The directionality of change scores

Cella et al (2002b) assessed cancer patients with the Functional Assessment of Cancer Therapy (FACT) and a Global Rating of Change. Patients were classified into five levels of change in HQoL based upon their responses to retrospective ratings of change after 2 months (sizably worse, minimally worse, no change, minimally better, and sizeably better). They found that the relationship between actual FACT change scores and retrospective ratings of change was modest but usually statistically significant. However, patients who reported global worsening of HQoL dimensions had considerably larger change scores than those reporting comparable global improvements.

In other words, relatively small gains in HQoL had substantial value for patients, while comparable declines seemed less meaningful. This finding is consistent with previous reports that patients adapt so as to minimize negative aspects of their condition.

As pointed out by Cella et al, factors such as adaptation/ response shift, dispositional optimism and the need for signs of clinical improvement may be contributing to the results, and require to be considered when interpreting the meaningfulness of change scores in HQoL questionnaires. One lesson may be that as adaptation works to *minimize* the impact of adverse states, and if a patient's global report is that their HQoL has deteriorated, it should generally be acted on (see Ch. 2).

Conclusion

There are two classes of method for interpreting HQoL change scores in a clinical situation. One is to relate scores to independent measures or anchors, such as patient global report or external events. Interpreting score differences based on doctors' views alone has been largely rejected. The second group is distribution-based, which entails translating score changes into SDs or SEMs. It would seem that both anchor-based and distribution-based methods have merit but neither is sufficient. Multiple strategies are desirable.

A further issue concerns patients' global reports and adaptation. Adaptation tends to suppress reports of worsening HQoL, so if the patient reports a change for the worse it should probably be acted on.

CROSS-CULTURAL APPLICATION ISSUES

There is a general need to consider whether measures are being validly applied as test populations deviate from the original groups upon which the tests were developed. English tests are being translated into European languages (e.g. see Keller et al 1998a) and Western tests are being steadily translated and offered for use in Asian cultures (e.g. see Chan-Yeung et al 2001, Thumboo et al 2002).

Tests are culture-laden

The use of Western tests in non-Western cultures seems particularly problematic. Collinge et al (2002) point out that what constitutes quality of life (QoL) is affected by an individual's beliefs, values, thoughts and attitudes; and cultures are instrumental in determining these. Culture may even influence the relationship between personality traits and well-being, e.g. extraversion seems correlated less strongly with pleasant affect in collectivistic nations than in individualistic nations (Diener & Lucas 2000).

Collinge et al (2002) suggested a range of issues require consideration when Western tools are used in non-Western cultures, including:

- *Beliefs about what constitutes QoL.* Quality of life may have a different meaning in non-Western cultures. For example, while Western ideals relate high QoL to successful self-improvement (school, work, study, etc.), Bengali culture places emphasis on role fulfillment: a girl may place greater value on fulfilling her role within the family as opposed to attending school.
- *QoL baselines and expectations.* Western expectations of lifetime employment or satisfactory leisure time do not represent ideals of a desirable life for people in countries dominated by civil war and famine. Bernheim (1999) described Rwanda where an immense number of people had lost their loved ones, their belongings, and been wounded themselves. Expectations and aspirations were necessarily different.
- *Communication style.* In some Asian cultures, overt expression of emotional distress is often rejected. Culturally sensitive measures of distress may be necessary.
- *Coping mechanisms.* Coping mechanisms may mediate subjective ratings of QoL. In many cultures, prayer is actively taught as a coping mechanism to promote a positive attitude to distress, and may mediate reports of QoL.

Trans-cultural tests could end up measuring little of importance

A related question arises with tests that have been specifically developed to be used in all cultures. These customarily seek out items that appear to function the same in all cultures, discarding items that exhibit differential item functioning or DIF.

There are likely to be problems in developing HQoL tests exclusively based on items that have a similar relationship to each other in all cultures examined. Salzberger (2000) pointed out the limitations of pursuing validity based on the internal structure of the construct but not related to criteria outside the construct, arguing that items showing differential item functioning should not be discarded blindly for they may be necessary to understand cultural differences. A construct (e.g. attitude to female education) may be able to be measured uniformly across cultures, but the significance of the construct may differ from one culture to another. If the measurement instrument is confined to the common denominator across cultures, the construct itself may become so narrowly defined that it severely threatens validity.

Salzberger argued that it is essential to determine exactly where cultures differ and where they do not. Items that are not suitable for cross-cultural comparisons should not be treated as distortions but seen as representing valuable information. As expressed by Salzberger, 'Disregarding intercultural validity may mean comparing apples and oranges while establishing inter-cultural validity means comparing apples and apples, or oranges and oranges. However, it might be the case that apples matter in one culture and oranges in another' (Salzberger 2000, p. 20).

The World Health Organization 'QoL' (WHOQoL) assessment represents one of the most prominent attempts to develop a pan-cultural measure (e.g. see Power et al 1999, Saxena et al 2001, Min et al 2002). Fox-Rushby & Parker (1995) argue that it too is likely to be flawed, because it proceeded from the view that there *are* universal dimensions of QoL and then framed questions from the perspective of educated middle class researchers that were likely to confirm this view. Fox-Rushby & Parker argued that all HQoL measures tend to be culture-full, not culture-free.

Where do 'cultures' end?

Concerns about instrument portability between different groups apply even when they share the same nationality and/or ethnicity. Stewart & Napoles-Springer (2000) point out that most HQoL measures were developed in non-minority, well-educated samples; and it cannot be assumed that such measures are conceptually and psychometrically equivalent in diverse sub-groups. They suggested that there has been little research exploring conceptual equivalence across US sub-groups, and that findings are inconsistent in the few studies that have been conducted. See also Barofsky (2000) and Wu (2000).

The argument can obviously be extended to each population sub-group and test purpose. Thus Eckerman (2000) has argued that there is a need for tests that are sensitive to gender; that QoL measures need to be gendered and differentiated to fully capture the diversity of women's and men's health experiences. In addition, the experiences and interests of older people are different (e.g. Kliempt et al 2000), as are those of younger people (see Ryan & Deci 2001).

Conclusion

Cultural values are likely to play an important role in QoL, and where cultural values differ, the importance of particular HQoL domains are also likely to differ. If care is not taken to recognize this, for some groups the relevant domains may not even be assessed.

MEASURING 'UTILITIES'
What are utilities?

As described in Chapter 1 under 'Tests Aiming to Measure Utility', health economists generally equate 'utility' with 'strength of preference'. However, there are a range of variations on this definition. Thus Feeny (2000) defines utility as 'a cardinal measure of the preference for, or desirability of, a specific level of health status or specific health outcome', while Lenert & Kaplan (2000) state that utilities are numeric measurements that reflect an individual's beliefs about the desirableness of a health condition, willingness to take risks to gain health benefits and preferences for time.

Traditionally, the measurement of utilities has been embedded in discussions regarding which is the appropriate measurement technique. The most common techniques have been the standard gamble, time tradeoff, and rating scale (Drummond et al 1987, see Box).

Note that as used in utility measurement, the rating scale (usually a visual analogue scale [VAS]) often employs death as one end-point. This has been periodically criticized on the grounds either that it distorts the nature of the scale (e.g. Carr-Hill 1992, referred to the 'quite legitimate refusal' of most normal people to rate death on the same scale as health states) or that there is a need for estimates corresponding to states worse than death (e.g. Sutherland et al 1983, Read et al 1984, Kind & Rosser 1988, Farsides & Dunlop 2001). Others have argued that the rating scale may not

Box 11.1 Traditional methods of measuring utilities

Drummond et al (1987) referred to the three most common methods for measuring health state utilities as: rating scale, standard gamble and time tradeoff.

A rating scale may consist of a line on a page with defined end-points, corresponding to a most preferred health state at one end and a least preferred health state at the other, which may or may not be 'Dead'. The subject selects a point on the scale deemed to be equivalent to the health state under investigation. If the 'healthy' end is 100, and the 'dead' end is 0, then the utility score can be read off in linear fashion.

The standard gamble is a much more complicated technique pursued by those who have chosen to adopt the approach to utility stated by Von Neumann & Morgenstern in 1953. It is concerned with estimating preferences under conditions of uncertainty. A subject will be presented with two alternatives: alternative one is a treatment with two possible outcomes – either the patient is returned to normal health and lives for t years (probability p), or the patient dies immediately (probability $1 - p$). Alternative two has the certain outcome of chronic state i for life (t years). Probability p is varied until the subject is indifferent between the two alternatives, at which point the required preference value for state i has been valued as p.

Note that the standard gamble has parallels to the situation that some patients can find themselves in – a treatment is offered as a means of staving off death from a terminal illness, but is known to be hazardous with an uncertain outcome. It does not follow, though, that this technique provides an accurate assessment of preference for health states. Richardson (1994, 1997) is a health economist who has strongly criticized the use of the standard gamble to gather utilities, arguing that its use is misconceived and anti-empirical, and that it measures the utility of gambling as much as the utility of health states.

There is evidence that risk is a multidimensional and cultural construct, with both individual and cultural differences: e.g. Bontempo et al (1997) found that subjects from Hong Kong and Thailand placed greater emphasis on the magnitude of losses, while subjects in the Netherlands and the USA emphasized the probabilities of losses (see also Kaplan et al 1993, Mellers et al 1998).

The Time tradeoff is a 'preference' method without uncertainty, and hence is much easier to apply than the standard gamble. Here, subjects are given a health state i for time t followed by death, and an alternative of complete health for time x ($x < t$). x is varied until the subject is indifferent between the two alternatives, at which point the preference for state i is determined as x/t.

be considered a true measure of utility, as it does not involve comparison against risk, time, or money (Tsevat 2000).

Whereas non-utility HQoL measures are principally concerned with assessing health states to monitor health and/or evaluate the effectiveness of healthcare interventions (individual or population-based), health utility measures are aimed at guiding decision making under uncertainty or under resource constraints. Hence they provide 'quality-adjustment factors' for the calculation of quality-adjusted life-years (QALYs) in decision analyses and cost-effectiveness analyses (Tsevat 2000 noted that health utility measures can also be used as end-points in clinical trials).

Utility theory may concern estimates of a single state or may be concerned with processes for aggregating a number of different utility dimensions. Multi-attribute utility theory is concerned with how to conduct such aggregations, e.g. via a weighted average of single-attribute utilities (e.g. Edwards & Fasolo 2001).

The consideration of future events

QALYs require active consideration of how to treat future health states (as do disability adjusted life years [DALYs], see Arnesen & Nord 1999). The issue is a highly complicated one.

As noted by Kaplan et al (1989), many health programmes affect the probability of occurrence of future dysfunction rather than altering current status. A person who is functional and asymptomatic today may be at risk of dying from heart disease in the future due to poor diet, etc. Health needs to include current and future components. Goodinson & Singleton (1989) noted that the use of 'satisfaction' in defining HQoL raised the issue of how to treat future satisfactions, e.g. should they be discounted.

Such events may or may not be apparent to the person involved. Individuals could be considered to be experiencing a lesser QoL by virtue of living in an area of major environmental pollution, with QoL seen to be diminished even if the effects of the pollution are not perceived or realized by those resident in the area. However, consciousness of possible future ill-health is likely also to affect *current* QoL (e.g. see Goodinson & Singleton 1989), and the complex process of adaptation (see Ch. 2).

Do preference measurement techniques predict outcomes?

A number of studies have sought to determine whether utility/preference measures provide valid estimates.

Saigal et al (2001) examined whether the utilities assigned by patients to possible complications of prostate cancer treatment predicted their actual treatment choice using multi-variety models. They estimated time tradeoff utility using time tradeoff, general

HQoL using the Rand 36-Item Health Survey, and prostate-targeted HQoL using the UCLA Prostate Cancer Index (PCI).

Saigal et al found that utility values elicited using time tradeoff were not significant predictors of treatment choice (while the prostate-targeted PCI HQoL measure was). They concluded that the time tradeoff method seemed to function poorly as a measure of patient preferences with localized prostate cancer, although they suggested it might be more effective if the morbidities were extremely severe and worth trading away some life span to avoid (e.g. blindness).

Cook et al (2001) examined the interval properties of utility models, which is an important issue if they are to be used for resource allocation. Cook et al applied the rating scale, standard gamble, and time tradeoff methods to assess descriptions of prostate-cancer-related health states using patients who had newly diagnosed, advanced prostate cancer, and plotted the boundaries between sub-ranges of the raw utilities and an equal-interval logit scale created using a Rasch model. They concluded that none of the utility scales seemed to function as interval-level scales.

However, this criticism could probably apply to most non-utility tests as well – see Chapter 8.

Will psychometrics be used to provide utility measures?

At one time, it was common for the standard gamble to be claimed as the 'gold standard' for utility measurement. Now there is a steady movement by health economists towards key elements of the psychometric perspective (although Torrance had earlier suggested that an alternative to assuming the necessary validity of the standard gamble was to measure the overall QoL associated with the health state and check that the utility measure thus formed was correlated with other trusted measures of HQoL; Torrance 1986).

Recently, Patrick & Chiang (2000b) stated that more attention should be given to particular application contexts and measurement objectives, and that the validation of utility measures is context-specific and no single elicitation process can be regarded as valid. Hawthorne et al (2001) proposed that no single multi-attribute utility instrument can claim to be the gold standard and that researchers should select an instrument sensitive to the health states they are investigating. Lenert & Kaplan (2000) suggest that future research must refine methods of eliciting utilities and identify sources of construct-irrelevant variability that reduce the validity of utility assessments. Nease (2000), along with Lenert & Kaplan (2000), concluded that it is not useful to think of an instrument as being valid or invalid and that the evidence must be assessed in support of its validity; and Brazier & Deverill (1999) set out an adaptation of the psychometric concepts of practicality, reliability and validity for assessing utility measures.

From the opposite perspective, psychometric health status measures have differed from utility measures in endeavouring to identify the elements responsible for a global HQoL score, and have favoured the patient as the source of information, while some utility theorists have advocated obtaining judgements from the general public. However, there seems no reason why a measure based on psychometric principles (entailing validity and reliability, pursued through empirical testing) cannot provide values for guiding resource allocation.

While such tests may not be based on decision making under uncertainty, this may be a good thing, given the evidence that decisions regarding imminent and future preferences may be both inaccurate and seemingly irrational (Redelmeier et al 1993, Loewenstein & Schkade 1997).

Conclusion

Health economists are become increasingly orientated towards empirical evaluation. There are increasing opportunities for health economists, psychometricians, and medical researchers to conduct collaborative research projects to create better tests and better healthcare decisions.

THE PROBLEM OF MISSING OR INCOMPLETE DATA

There is a growing literature on the difficulties posed by missing or incomplete HQoL data, the problems of which can be substantial, particularly in cancer clinical trials.

The problem is particularly serious as it cannot be assumed that the data are missing at random (Fairclough et al 1998, Moinpour et al 2000), i.e. patients who fail to complete HQoL forms will tend to have lower HQoL (Coates & Gebski 1998, Simes et al 1998).

Prevention of missing data

Following an extensive review of papers relevant to the area, Bernhard et al (1998) made a series of recommendations on how to minimize missing data. The following presents a summary of the means they identified, addressing methodological, logistical/administrative and patient-related factors.

Methodological factors

Data loss can be minimized by:

- Careful definition of the minimum amount of, and timing of data, and what degree of deviation from exact timing is acceptable.
- Special attention to the baseline assessment, as complete data are essential and the baseline assessment may be a powerful predictor of subsequent submission rates.
- Assessing respondent burden carefully, as questionnaire completion will become more difficult if patients' conditions deteriorate, and in almost all cancer trials with HQoL endpoints, there is a decrease of questionnaire submission rates over time.
- Use of shorter instruments, if possible.

Logistical and administrative factors

Data loss can be minimized by:

- Adequately funding HQoL data management (essential).
- Mailing reminders concerning outstanding questionnaires directly to patients (increasing response rate by up to 50%).
- Completing the questionnaire by telephone, or use of the telephone if mail-out method is unsuccessful (this is more reliable and convenient for the patients, but cost-intensive).
- Telephoning patients just before the questionnaires are sent out, and if the questionnaires are not returned within 2 weeks, sending a reminder letter (this is reported to result in submission rates of not less than 87% at 3 year follow-up).
- Randomizing into the trial only patients who complete a baseline measure (this is reported to lead to 95% compliance); also pre-trial workshops to train nurses and data managers in collecting HQoL data.

- Commitment by staff – the clinician and nurse or data manager involved in the trial must be committed to the HQoL component, with their support secured prior to initiating the study and continuously reinforced.
- Maintaining quality control – ensuring that questionnaires are given to the patient, that the right questionnaires are given, and that questionnaires are administered at the right time, etc.
- Taking staff changes into account, as accrual and follow-up in cancer clinical trials can take years (continuous instruction is needed as part of trial coordination and monitoring).

Bernhard et al (1998) observed that questionnaire submission rates in multi-centre trials depended more on the institution and the attitude of the treating physician, than the clinical or sociodemographic characteristics of the individual patient.

Patient-related factors

Data loss can be minimized by:

- Staff recognizing the need to encourage and motivate patients to complete the questionnaire, especially if there are frequent repeat assessments.
- Use of information on health status in advanced disease trials where some patients will be too ill to complete the questionnaire, to interpret whether any treatment effects were related to missing QoL data; proxies may also be valuable when there are no other QoL data.
- Particularly supporting elderly patients and those with lower education and poorer physical functioning.
- Recognizing that the effect of patient characteristics on missing data can be quite different at baseline versus during treatment.
- Realizing that the capacity of patients to complete HQoL forms may be directly affected by the study intervention.
- Recognizing that cultural restrictions can cause patient reluctance to participate (assessment of sensitive issues may not be feasible where such questions would be considered an invasion of privacy).

In conclusion, Bernhard et al (1998) observed that there is broad consensus that patient-related factors are much less of a problem than logistical and administrative problems, particularly staff oversights, and that a dedicated and adequately resourced study co-ordinator with good interpersonal skills can prevent most of the avoidable sources of missing data.

Dealing with missing data

Fayers et al (1998) examined the widely practiced approach of imputation using the mean of all observed items in the same sub-scale. They showed that this may be an inappropriate method for many of the items in QoL questionnaires and would result in biased or misleading estimates, and proposed a checklist for examining the adequacy of simple imputation as well as some alternative procedures.

Simes et al (1998) proposed that clinical trials should include the collection of auxiliary health status information to allow imputing missing QoL data based on such data.

Troxel et al (1998) described different types of missing data in cancer clinical trials and ways of assessing and testing missing data mechanisms. They described the use of graphical displays to document the extent of the missing data problem and its impact on interpretation of results, and discussed statistical methods used to analyze repeated measures with their ability to handle missing data.

The practice of imputation, using the mean of all observed items in the same sub-scale when analyzing data from clinical trials, was discussed by Fayers et al (1998). They argued this may be an inappropriate method for many of the items in QoL questionnaires, would result in biased or misleading estimates, and offer a checklist for examining the adequacy of simple imputation and some alternative procedures. Simes et al (1998) discussed the value of collecting auxiliary health status information in clinical trials to allow estimation of missing QoL data.

Curran et al (1998) provided an overview of methods for analyzing incomplete longitudinal QoL data, with the methods classified by the conditions the data need to meet.

Reporting requirements for missing data

Bernhard et al (1998) stated that investigators have an obligation to provide enough information to allow the reader to assess the quality of the study and provided a sample missing data reporting form to be completed at each assessment time for every patient. They maintained that three questions should be able to be answered:

1. How many missing data are there?
2. Why were the data missing?
3. How will the missing data affect the interpretation of the study results?

Bernhard et al (1998) recommended that treatment group differences in submission rates be compared (when applicable), and that examination of other patient and institution-related factors affecting submission rates be conducted to further classify the reasons for missing data and identify differences between patients with and without data (e.g. by comparing characteristics of responders and non-responders, or using logistic regression models to evaluate the association between submission rates and selected factors).

They further recommended that the quality of completed questionnaire be evaluated in terms of item-response rates, so as to identify items that may have caused particular problems for patients and to help evaluate how missing items will affect the calculation of summated scales.

Machin & Weeden (1998) may be consulted for a step-by-step approach to presentation of HQoL data, with an emphasis on examining data graphically before analysis and to facilitate interpretation in the final report.

Conclusion

Since most HQoL measurements require patient self-report, it is usually not possible to rectify missing data. Unfortunately, such data are generally not 'missing at random' and cannot be ignored without introducing bias.

Several approaches to the analysis of partly missing data are available, but none is entirely satisfactory. Prevention of missing data is the best approach.

As concluded by Curran et al (1998, p. 707), 'Sufficient care and attention should be taken at the design stage of a study to ensure an adequate infrastructure, including appropriate personnel and material to carry out the study. No matter how well the analysis is thought out and how accurate assumptions are about missing data mechanisms, inferences in the presence of incomplete data are not as convincing as inferences based on a complete data set'.

The journal *Statistics in Medicine* (vol. 17, pp. 511–1998) provided a special supplement reporting on papers from an international conference on missing HQoL data in cancer clinical trials. The supplement extensively explored the issues and may be usefully consulted by those involved with measuring HQoL in cancer trials.

DYNAMIC MEASURES

Most patient-based measures of health status (HQoL, functional status, etc.) offer characterizations or estimates of the current state of the patient or client. However, tests that assess health-related behaviours may go beyond description to outcome prevention.

These *dynamic measures*, so-called because they are based on patients being active agents in their health state, are expressions of what Wyrwich & Wolinsky (2000; after Kirshner & Guyatt 1985) termed predictive instruments, i.e. instruments which identify individuals who have or will develop specific conditions.

In this context, to achieve the potential of patient-based measures, it is necessary to recognize that:

- health states are the results of many interactions
- the person is an active agent in their current and future health state
- 'healthcare structure and processes' include not just hospitals and healthcare workers but community-based and orientated programmes
- the 'patient' operates in a social milieu, with family and others involved, both as care givers and as people who may experience a decline in their own health because of the patient's state.

This approach recognizes that health outcomes are the result of a dynamic system, as represented in Figure 11.1.

Measures that actively recognize and incorporate this broad context have the potential to reveal what a person's health state is, why it is so, and identify *where and how to intervene* to more effectively and efficiently improve the health state.

Such tests represent theories of how health-related behaviours lead to or entrench illnesses. For example, behavioural research has helped identify psychosocial variables associated with cancer risk behaviours (Schneiderman et al 2001). Such information can play a vital role in tests that identify at-risk individuals and distinguish

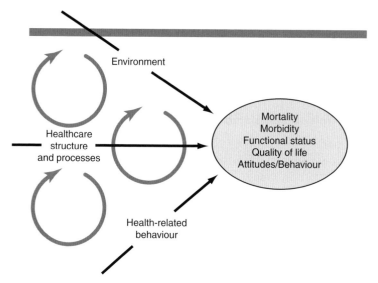

Figure 11.1   What is the outcome and why?

the responsible variables. These tests have the potential for early identification and/or prevention of a range of health conditions.

The Asthma Medication Adherence Questionnaire

The Asthma Medication Adherence Questionnaire (AMAQ) is a member of this new breed, an instrument developed by the author (supported by GlaxoSmithKline) for estimating patient adherence with asthma preventer medication (O'Connor et al 2000). AMAQ aimed to identify the self-reported attitudes and behaviours associated with non-adherence and lay them out in a predictive model.

Based on the literature, and discussions with healthcare professionals and patients, variables potentially predictive of adherence were first identified (e.g. 'relationship with doctor'). These variables acted as predictors of (confidential) quantitative reports of adherence. A predictive model was then formed using multiple regression. The initial form of AMAQ was made up of questions relating to non-adherent behaviours, e.g. 'At least once a month I have stopped taking my medication for at least 3 days'; relationship with doctor, e.g. 'My doctor gives me plenty of time and is warm and understanding'; and degree of sleeplessness, 'Awoke at night or couldn't get to sleep due to asthma'.

The AMAQ was the first instrument to estimate asthma-medication adherence based on patients' reports of their attitudes and behaviours. It offered a method for estimating or predicting adherence under conditions where direct measurement was unreliable or not possible.

Application of dynamic models

Dynamic models have application to a range of conditions, such as diabetes, child abuse, and carer burden. Such models are likely to need to incorporate a broad range of variables, such as attitudes to illness, availability of appropriate treatments, nutrition, peer influences, relationship with the health system, specific cultural factors, socio-economic status, etc.

There would seem to be great potential for moving from the current situation of patient-centred measures as descriptions (HQoL), to instruments playing diagnostic roles identifying areas of concern to patients (and possibly new treatments), to models of 'dynamic' states based on health-related behaviours that can identify possible future health states.

As proposed in a recent review conducted for the US Agency for Health Care Policy and Research (AHCPR 1999) there is a need to move from a 'tool-using' culture to a 'problem solving' culture, for which the primary objective is developing an empirical science of clinical improvement, i.e. an emphasis on improvement over assessment.

SUMMARY AND CONCLUSIONS

Among the issues that need to be resolved for the most effective application of patient-centred health outcome measures are the following:

Interpreting quality of life scores for individual patients

For HQoL measures to be incorporated effectively into clinical practice, methods for interpreting HQoL change scores in a clinical situation are required.

Current approaches are to relate scores to independent measures or 'anchors' (e.g. patient global report, or external events) in terms of number of MCIDs or 'minimal clinical importance differences', or to assess changes in score in terms of numbers of standard deviation or standard error units (e.g. 'moderate change' when equivalent to 0.5 standard deviations). At the current time it would seem that both anchor-based and distribution-based methods have merit but neither is sufficient, and that multiple strategies are desirable.

A further issue concerns adaptation. Adaptation tends to suppress reports of worsening HQoL, so patient's reports of a change need to be considered carefully.

Cross-cultural application issues

There is a general need to consider whether measures are being validly applied as test populations deviate from the original groups upon which the tests were developed (the use of Western tests in non-Western cultures seems particularly problematic).

What constitutes 'quality of life' is affected by an individual's beliefs and values, and is largely culturally determined.

Moreover, items that may be considered unsuitable to cross-cultural comparisons through exhibiting 'differential item functioning' should *not* be eliminated from further consideration, as they may represent essential cultural distinctions and convey valuable information.

Care is needed to recognize this, otherwise HQoL measures may be developed or selected that fail to assess what for some cultural (or sub-cultural) groups are the most important domains.

Measuring 'utilities'

There currently seems to be a movement by health economists towards key elements of the psychometric perspective, deviating from the once dominant notion that use of a particular utility-elicitation method would automatically produce the correct values (e.g. 'the standard gamble' technique). It seems increasingly accepted that a 'utility' instrument is not valid or invalid, but that evidence must be gathered to assess its degree of practicality, reliability and validity.

Evidence that decisions regarding imminent and future preferences may be both inaccurate and seemingly irrational is likely to encourage this movement, the earlier tendency to rely on general members of the public for utilities of illness states being increasingly discredited.

There are growing opportunities for health economists, psychometricians, and medical researchers to collaborate to create tests that can better guide resource allocation decisions and healthcare decisions generally.

The problem of missing or incomplete data

There can be considerable difficulties posed by missing or incomplete HQoL data. The problem is particularly serious in cancer clinical trials as it cannot be assumed that the data are missing at random, i.e. it is the most ill patients for whom data are not forthcoming. The data are not 'missing at random' and cannot be ignored without introducing bias.

Since most HQoL measurements require patient self-report, it is usually not possible to replace missing data. While several approaches to the analysis of partly missing data are available, none is entirely satisfactory. Ultimately, prevention of missing data is the best approach. Care and attention is needed at the design stage to ensure adequate infrastructure, appropriate personnel, and careful quality control, to minimize data loss.

Conclusions when there are incomplete data are never as convincing as when data are complete.

Dynamic measures: measuring health-related behaviour to prevent future outcomes

Most patient-centred measures of health status (HQoL, functional status, etc.) offer characterizations or estimates of the current state of the patient or client. There is a need to overcome the static approach to QoL assessment embodied by such tests, to recognize that people are active participants in their own future health.

Tests that assess health-related behaviours may go beyond description to outcome prevention. Developing tests that represent 'dynamic models' of the attitudes and behaviours associated with particular chronic illnesses may both identify individuals at risk and reveal the behaviours and/or attitudes that could be targeted to prevent such illnesses.

Appendices

Examples of common item types

GUTTMAN SCALE

'Table 6: Ability to manipulate objects for work, over the next 2 years'
This Table measures the impact of the applicant's impairment upon their ability to manipulate everyday and work objects.

0   While may experience some discomfort, able to manipulate objects freely.

30 Some reduction in dexterity and/or speed of manipulation of objects as a result of impairment(s), e.g. difficulty smoothly placing key in lock, teaspoon of sugar in coffee, but able to turn door handles, manipulate money, write, use a keyboard, use hand tools, etc.

75 Substantially diminished dexterity and/or speed of manipulation as a result of impairment(s), unable to turn door handles and/or manipulate money, write, use a keyboard, use hand tools, etc.

LIKERT SCALE

'Please indicate the extent to which the following statements reflect your views/experience of your scheduled medication over the last 3 months. (Please tick one box only for each statement.)
Overall, my scheduled medication:

	Strongly disagree	Disagree	Neither agree nor disagree	Agree	Strongly agree
a. Makes me feel better				✔	

VISUAL ANALOGUE SCALE

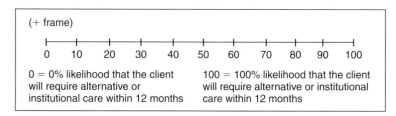

(+ frame)

|---+---+---+---+---+---+---+---+---+---|
0   10   20   30   40   50   60   70   80   90   100

0 = 0% likelihood that the client will require alternative or institutional care within 12 months

100 = 100% likelihood that the client will require alternative or institutional care within 12 months

DICHOTOMOUS ITEM

(+ frame)

'I isolate myself as much as I can from the rest of my family'   Yes/No

Internet resources

The following lists some of the internet sites related to health-related quality of life (HQoL) measurement that may be of use. The resources listed are by no means exhaustive, and cannot be assumed to be current: internet resources tend to be in a state of continual change and the links may or may not be active when access is sought.

SOCIETIES RELATED TO QUALITY OF LIFE

International Society for Quality of Life Research (ISOQOL), the society most concerned with the scientific study of quality of life relevant to health and healthcare
http://www.isoqol.org/

International Society for Quality of Life Studies
http://www.cob.vt.edu/market/isqols/

Society for Medical Decision Making
http://www.smdm.org/main.html

International Health Economics Association
http://healtheconomics.org/cgibin/WebObjects/ihea

Drug Information Association
http://www.diahome.org/docs/index.cfm

International Society for Pharmacoeconomics and Outcomes Research (ISPOR)
www.ispor.org

QUALITY OF LIFE AND/OR HEALTH ECONOMICS SITES PROVIDING USEFUL LINKS

Quality of Life Instruments Database (QOLID)
http://www.qolid.org/

MAPI Research Institute
www.mapi-research-inst.com

Medical Outcomes Trust (access to SF-36)
http://www.outcomes-trust.org/instruments.htm

RAND Health
www.rand.org/health_area

Trent Research Information Access Gateway – Health Economics (TRIAGE)
http://www.shef.ac.uk/~scharr/triage/index/health.htm

REES France Health Evaluation Network
http://www.rees-france.com/sites.htm

SNOF LA QUALITÉ DE VIE
http://www.snof.org/melody/interface/qualite/qualite.php?rubrique = liens

Evaluación Clinica Y Economica de Medicamentos
http://www.farmacoeconomia.com/CalidadDeVida/CalidadDeVidaInstrument
osNew.htm

ON-LINE STATISTICAL TEXTS

StatSoft Inc. Electronic Statistics Textbook
http://www.statsoft.com/textbook/stathome.html

Introductory Statistics: Concepts, Models, and Applications
David W. Stockburger, Southwest Missouri State University
http://www.psychstat.smsu.edu/introbook/sbk00.htm

Multivariate Statistics: Concepts, Models, and Applications
David W. Stockburger, Southwest Missouri State University
http://www.psychstat.smsu.edu/multibook/mlt00.htm

Bill Trochim's Social Research Methods
http://trochim.human.cornell.edu/

MEDICAL JOURNALS

The principal databases concerned with HQoL measurement are MEDLINE and
PsycINFO. Further relevant material may be located elsewhere, e.g. via health
economics sources.

PubMed, a service of the National Library of Medicine, includes over 14 million
citations for biomedical articles back to the 1950s. These citations are from
MEDLINE and additional life science journals. PubMed includes links to many
sites providing full text articles and other related resources. See: http://www.
ncbi.nlm.nih.gov/entrez/query.fcgi

The British Medical Journal (BMJ) at www.bmj.com is also available free on-line,
and includes a substantial proportion of HQoL articles.

PsycINFO is a database of psychological literature from the 1800s to the present.
See: http://www.apa.org/psycinfo/

MISCELLANEOUS

The Institute for Objective Measurement provides a large amount of information
concerning Modern Test Theory from the perspective of the Rasch Model, including the Rasch Measurement Transactions. See: http://www.rasch.org/

Rod O'Connor & Associates, includes an 80 page review of issues in measuring
HQoL. See: http://www.rodoconnorassoc.com

References

Aaronson N, Alonso J, Burnam A et al 2002 Assessing health status and quality-of-life instruments: attributes and review criteria. Quality of Life Research 11:193–205

Adang E M M, Kootstra G, van Hoeff J P et al 1998 Do retrospective and prospective quality of life assessments differ for pancreas-kidney transplant recipients? Transplant International 11:11–15

AERA, APA, NCME 1999 Standards for educational and psychological testing. American Educational Research Association, American Psychological Association and National Council on Measurement in Education

AHCPR 1999 The outcome of outcomes research at AHCPR: final report. Summary. Agency for Health Care Policy and Research, Rockville, MD. Available: http://www.ahrq.gov/clinic/outcosum.htm Downloaded September 1999

Anastasi A 1986 Evolving concepts of test validation. Annual Review of Psychology 37:1–15

Anastasi A 1990 Psychological testing, 6th edn. MacMillan Publishing Company, New York

Anastasi A, Urbina S 1997 Psychological testing, 7th edn. Prentice Hall Inc., Upper Saddle River, NJ

Anderson N H 1976 How functional measurement can yield validated interval scales of mental attitudes. Journal of Applied Psychology 61(6):677–692

Andrich D 1982 An index of person separation in latent trait theory, the traditional KR-20 Index, and the Guttman scale response pattern. Education Research and Perspectives 9(1):95–104

Ariely D 1998 Combining experiences over time: the effects of duration, intensity changes and on-line measurements of retrospective pain evaluations. Journal of Behavioural Decision Making 11:19–45

Arnesen T, Nord E 1999 The value of DALY life: problems with ethics and validity of disability adjusted life years. British Medical Journal 319:1423–1425

Awad A G, Voruganti L N, Heslegrave R J 1997 Measuring quality of life in patients with schizophrenia. Pharmacoeconomics 11(1):32–47

Badia X, Prieto L, Roset M et al 2002 Development of a short osteoporosis quality of life questionnaire by equating items from two existing instruments. Journal of Clinical Epidemiology 55:32–40

Baker F B 2001 The Basics of item response theory, 2nd edn. Published by the ERIC Clearinghouse on Assessment and Evaluation, USA

Balaban D J, Sagi P C, Goldfarb N I et al 1986 Weights for scoring the quality of well being instrument among rheumatoid arthritics. Medical Care 24:973–980

Bar-On D, Lazar A, Amir M 2000 Quantitative assessment of response shift in QOL research. Social Indicators Research 49(1):37–49

Barofsky I 2000 The role of cognitive equivalence in studies of health-related quality-of-life assessments. Medical Care 38(9, suppl):II 125–129

Bennett S J, Oldridge N B, Eckert G J et al 2002 Discriminant properties of commonly used quality of life measures in heart failure. Quality of Life Research 11:349–359

Bergner M 1989 Quality of life, health status, and clinical research. Medical Care 27:S148–S156

Bergner M, Bobbitt R, Kressel S et al 1976a The sickness impact profile: conceptual foundations and methodology for the development of a health status measure. International Journal of Health Services 6:393–415

Bergner M, Bobbitt R, Pollard W et al 1976b The sickness impact profile: validation of a health status measure. Medical Care XIV:57–67

Bergner M, Bobbitt R A, Carter W B et al 1981 The sickness impact profile: development and final revision of a health status measure. Medical Care XIX:787–805

Bernhard J, Cella D F, Coates A S et al 1998 Missing quality of life data in cancer clinical trials: serious problems and challenges. Statistics in Medicine 17:517–532

Bernheim J L 1999 How to get serious answers to the serious question: 'How have you been?': subjective quality of life (QoL) as an individual experiential emergent construct. Bioethics 13(3–4):272–287

Berzon R A, Leplège A P, Lohr K N et al 1997 Summary and recommendations for future research. Quality of Life Research 6:601–605

Bezjak A, Ng P, Skeel R et al 2001 Oncologists' use of quality of life information results of a survey of Eastern Cooperative Oncology Group physicians. Quality of Life Research 10:1–13

Birbeck G L, Kim S, Hays R D et al 2000 Quality of life measures in epilepsy. How well can they detect change over time? Neurology 54:1822–1827

Bjorner J B, Ware J E, Kosinski M 2003 The potential synergy between cognitive models and modern psychometric models. Quality of Life Research 12:261–274

Bollen K A 2002 Latent variables in psychology and the social sciences. Annual Review of Psychology 53:605–634

Bond T G, Fox C M 2001 Applying the Rasch model: fundamental measurement in the human sciences. Lawrence Erlbaum Associates, London

Bonsignore M, Barkow K, Jessen F et al 2001 Validity of the five-item WHO Well-Being Index (WHO-5) in an elderly population. European Archives of Psychiatry and Clinical Neuroscience 251(suppl 2):II/27–II/31

Bontempo R N, Bottom W P, Weber E U 1997 Cross-cultural differences in risk perception: a model-based approach. Risk Analysis 17:479–488

Bottomley A 2002 The cancer patient and quality of life. The Oncologist 7:120–125

Bowling A 1997 Measuring health: a review of quality of life measurement scales, 2nd edn. Open University Press, Buckingham

Boyle M H, Torrance G W, Sinclair J C et al 1983 Economic evaluation of neonatal intensive care of very-low-birth-weight infants. New England Journal of Medicine 308:1330–1337

Brazier J, Deverill M 1999 A checklist for judging preference-based measures of health related quality of life: learning from psychometrics. Health Economics 8(1):41–51

Breetvelt I S, Van Dam F S 1991 Under reporting by cancer patients: the case of response-shift. Social Science and Medicine 32(9):981–987

Brickman P, Coates D, Janoff-Bulman R 1978 Lottery winners and accident victims: is happiness relative? Journal of Personality and Social Psychology 37:917–927

Brooks R 1996 EuroQoL: the current state of play. Health Policy 37:53–72

Brooks R G 1991 Health status and quality of life measurement: issues and developments. The Swedish Institute for Health Economics, IHE, Lund

Calman K C 1984 Quality of life in cancer patients – an hypothesis. Journal of Medical Ethics 10(3):124–127

Campbell A 1981 The sense of well-being in America. McGraw-Hill, New York

Campbell D T, Fiske D W 1959 Convergent and discriminant validation by the multitrait – multimethod matrix. Psychological Bulletin 56:81–105

Carlsson M, Hamrin E 2002 Evaluation of the life satisfaction questionnaire (LSQ) using structural equation modelling (SEM). Quality of Life Research 11:415–425

Caro J J, Caro I, Caro J et al 2001 Does electronic implementation of questionnaires used in asthma alter responses compared to paper implementation? Quality of Life Research 10:683–691

Carr A J, Higginson I J 2001 Measuring quality of life: are quality of life measures patient centered? British Medical Journal 322:1357–1360

Carr A J, Gibson B, Robinson P G 2001 Measuring quality of life: is quality of life determined by expectations or experience? British Medical Journal 322:1240–1243

Carr-Hill R A 1992 Health related quality of life measurement – Euro style. Health Policy 20(3):321–328, discussion 329–332

Carter W B, Bobbitt R A, Bergner M et al 1976 Validation of an interval scaling: the sickness impact profile. Health Services Research 11:516–528

Cella D, Chang C-H 2000 A discussion of item response theory and its applications in health status assessment. Medical Care 38(9, suppl):II 66–72

Cella D, Bullinger M, Scott C et al 2002a Group vs individual approaches to understanding the clinical significance of differences or changes in quality of life. Source Mayo Clinic Proceedings 77(4):384–392

Cella D, Hahn E A, Dineen K 2002b Meaningful change in cancer-specific quality of life scores: differences between improvement and worsening. Quality of Life Research 11(3):207–221

Chan-Yeung M, Law B, Sheung S Y et al 2001 Internal consistency, reproducibility, responsiveness, and construct validity of the Chinese (HK) version of the asthma quality of life questionnaire. Quality of Life Research 10:723–730

Chang V T, Thaler H T, Polyak T A et al 1998 Quality of life and survival. The role of multidimensional symptom assessment. Cancer 83(1):173–179

Christensen-Szalanski J J 1984 Discount functions and the measurement of patients' values. Women's decisions during childbirth. Medical Decision Making 4(1):47–58

Clancy C M, Eisenberg J M 1998 Measuring the end results of health care. Science 282:245–246

Clancy C M, Lipscomb J 2000 From the sponsors. Medical Care 38(9, suppl) II:II-2

Coates A, Gebski V 1998 Quality of life studies of the Australian New Zealand Breast Cancer Trials Group: approaches to missing data. Statistics in Medicine (5–7):533–540

Cohen J 1968 Multiple regression as a general data analysis system. Psychological Bulletin 70:426–443

Cohen G, Forbes J, Garraway M 1996 Can different patient satisfaction survey methods yield consistent results? Comparison of three surveys. British Medical Journal 313:841–844

Cohen R J, Swerdlik M E 1999 Psychological testing and assessment: an introduction to tests and measurement, 4th edn. Mayfield Publishing Company, London

Collinge A, Rudell K, Bhui K 2002 Quality of life assessment in non-Western cultures. International Review of Psychiatry 14:212–218

Cook K F, Ashton C M, Byrne M M et al 2001 A psychometric analysis of the measurement level of the rating scale, time trade-off, and standard gamble. Social Science and Medicine 53:1275–1285

Coyne K, Revicki D, Hunt T et al 2002 Psychometric validation of an overactive bladder symptom and health-related quality of life questionnaire: The OAB-q. Quality of Life Research 11:563–574

Cramer J A 1999 Quality of life assessment in clinical practice. Neurology 53(5, suppl 2):S49–52

Crocker L M, Algina J 1986 Introduction to classical and modern test theory. Holt, Rinehart and Winston, New York

Cronbach L J 1971 Test validation. In: Thorndike RL (ed) Educational measurement, 2nd edn. American Council on Education, Washington

Crowley S L, Fan X 1997 Structural equation modeling: basic concepts and applications in personality assessment research. Journal of Personality Assessment 68(3):508–531

Croyle R T, Uretsky M B 1987 Effects of mood on self-appraisal of health status. Health Psychology 6:239–253

Cummins R A 2000 Objective and subjective quality of life: an interactive model. Social Indicators Research 52:55–72

Curran D, Molenburghs G, Fayers P M et al 1998 Incomplete quality of life data in randomized trials: missing forms. Statistics in Medicine 17:697–709

Damiano A M 1996 The sickness impact profile. In: Spilker B (ed) Quality of life and pharmacoeconomics in clinical trials, 2nd edn. Lippincott-Raven Publishers, Philadelphia, pp. 306–322

Danner D D, Snowdon D A, Friesen W V 2001 Positive emotions in early life and longevity: findings from the nun study. Journal of Personality and Social Psychology 80:804–813

Dempster M, Donnelly M, Fitzsimons D 2002 Generic, disease-specific and individualised approaches to measuring health-related quality of life among people with heart disease – a comparative analysis. Psychology and Health 17(4):447–457

Desselle S P, Vaughan M, Faria T 2002 Creating a performance appraisal template for pharmacy technicians using the method of equal-appearing intervals. Journal of the American Pharmaceutical Association 42(5):768–779

Detmar S B, Aaronson N K 1998 Quality of life assessment in daily clinical oncology practice: a feasibility study. European Journal of Cancer 34:1181–1186

Devins G M, Dion R, Pelletier L G et al 2001 Structure of lifestyle disruptions in chronic disease. A confirmatory factor analysis of the illness intrusiveness ratings scale. Medical Care 39(10):1097–1104

Deyo R A, Patrick L P 1989 Barriers to the use of health status measures in clinical investigation, patient care, and policy research. Medical Care 27(3, suppl):S254–268

Dickson H G, Köhler F 1996 The multi-dimensionality of the FIM motor items precludes an interval scaling using Rasch analysis. Scandinavian Journal of Rehabilitation Medicine 26:159–162

Diener E 1984 Subjective well-being. Psychological Bulletin 45:542–575

Diener E, Diener M 1995 Cross-cultural correlates of life satisfaction and self-esteem. Journal of Personality and Social Psychology 68:653–663

Diener E, Lucas R E 2000 Subjective emotional well-being. In: Lewis M, Haviland J M (eds) Handbook of emotions, 2nd edn. Guilford, New York pp. 325–337

Diener E, Suh E M, Lucas R E et al 1999 Subjective well-being: three decades of progress. Psychological Bulletin 125:276–302

Dijkers M P, Whiteneck G, El-Jaroudi R 2000 Measures of social outcomes in disability research. Archives of Physical Medicine and Rehabilitation 81(12, suppl 2):S63–80

Donaldson L 2003 Expert patients usher in a new era of opportunity for the NHS. British Medical Journal 326:1279–1280

Donovan K, Sanson-Fisher R W, Redman S 1989 Measuring quality of life in cancer patients. Journal of Clinical Oncology 7:959–968

Drummond M, Stoddart G, Torrance G 1987 Methods for the economic evaluation of health care programmes. Oxford Medical Publications, Oxford University Press

Ebel R L 1961 Must all tests be valid? American Psychologist 16:640–647

Ebrahim S 1995 Clinical and public health perspectives and applications of health-related quality of life measurement. Social Science and Medicine 41(10):1383–1394

Eckerman L 2000 Gendering indicators of health and well-being: is quality of life gender neutral? Social Indicators Research 52(1):29–54

Edwards W, Fasolo B 2001 Decision technology. Annual Review of Psychology 52:581–606

Embretson S 1996 The new rules of measurement. Psychological Assessment 8(4):341–349

Epstein A M, Hall J A, Tognetti J et al 1989 Using proxies to evaluate quality of life. Medical Care 27(3):S91–S98

Epstein R S, Lydick E 1995 Quality of life assessment: a pharmaceutical industry perspective. In: Dimsdale J E, Baum A (eds) Quality of life in behavioural medicine research. Erlbaum Associates, New York, NY

Erickson P 2000 Assessment of the evaluative properties of health status instruments. Medical Care 38(9, suppl):II 95–101

EuroQoL Group 1990 EuroQol – a new facility for the measurement of health-related quality of life. Health Policy 16:199–208

Eyfuth K 1972 'Scaling'. In: Eysenck H J, Arnold W J, Meili R (eds) Encyclopaedia of psychology. Fontana/Collins

Fahey T, Griffiths S, Peters T J 1995 Evidence based purchasing: understanding results of clinical trials and systematic reviews. British Medical Journal 311:1056–1059

Fairclough D L, Peterson H F, Chang V 1998 Why are missing quality of life data a problem in clinical trials of cancer therapy? Statistics in Medicine 17(5–7):667–677

Fakhoury W K H, Priebe S 2002 Subjective quality of life: its association with other constructs. International Review of Psychiatry 14:219–224

Fan X 1998 Item response theory and classical test theory: an empirical comparison of their item/person statistics. Educational and Psychological Measurement 58(3):357

Farsides B, Dunlop R J 2001 Is there such a thing as a life not worth living? British Medical Journal 322(7300):1481–1483

Fayers P M, Curran D, Machin D 1998 Incomplete quality of life data in randomized trials: missing items. Statistics in Medicine 17(5–7):679–696

Feeny D 2000 A utility approach to the assessment of health-related quality of life. Medical Care 38(9, suppl):II 151–154

Feeny D H, Torrance G W 1989 Incorporating utility-based quality-of-life assessment measures in clinical trials. Medical Care 27(3):S190–S204

Feeny D, Juniper E F, Ferrie P J et al 1998 Why not just ask the kids? Health-related quality of life in children with asthma. In: Drotar D (ed) Measuring health-related quality of life in children and adolescents: implications for research and practice. Lawrence Erlbaum Associates, Inc., London, pp. 171–185

Feinstein A R 1999 Multi-item 'instruments' vs Virginia Apgar's principles of clinimetrics. Archives of Internal Medicine 159(2):125–128

Ferguson G A 1966 Statistical analysis in psychology and education, 2nd edn. McGraw Hill, London

Fox-Rushby J, Parker M 1995 Culture and the measurement of health-related quality of life. European Review of Applied Psychology 45(4):257–263

Frary R B 1996a Hints for designing effective questionnaires. Practical assessment, research and evaluation 5(3). Online. Available: http://ericae.net/pare/getvn.asp?v=5&n=3

Frary R B 1996b Brief guide to questionnaire development. ERIC Clearinghouse on Assessment and Evaluation, Washington, DC

Gardner D G, Cummings L L, Dunham R B et al 1998 Single-item versus multiple-item measurement scales: an empirical comparison. Educational and Psychological Measurement 58(i6):898(1)

Gardner K, Chapple A 1999 Barriers to referral in patients with angina: qualitative study. British Medical Journal 319:418–421

Garratt A, Schmidt L, Mackintosh A et al 2002 Quality of life measurement: bibliographic study of patient assessed health outcomes measures. British Medical Journal 24:1417

Gescheider G A 1988 Psychophysical scaling. Annual Review of Psychology 39:169–200

Giesler R B, Ashton C M, Brody B, Byrne M M et al 1999 Assessing the performance of utility techniques in the absence of a gold standard. Medical Care 37(6):580–588

Gill T M, Feinstein A R 1994 A critical appraisal of the quality-of-life measurements. JAMA 272:619–626

Goodinson S M, Singleton J 1989 Quality of life: a critical review of current concepts, measures, and their clinical implications. International Journal of Nursing Studies 6(4):327–341

Goodwin L D 2002 Changing conceptions of measurement validity: an update on the new standards. Journal of Nursing Education 41(3):100–106

Gudex C 1986 QALY's, and their use by the health service. Discussion Paper 20, Centre for Health Economics, University of York

Guyatt G H 2000 Making sense of quality-of-life data. Medical Care 38(9, suppl):II 175–179

Guyatt G H, Osoba D, Wu A W et al 2002 Clinical Significance Consensus Meeting Group. Methods to explain the clinical significance of health status measures. Mayo Clinic Proceedings 77(4):371–383

Haas B K 1999 Clarification and integration of similar quality of life concepts. Image – the Journal of Nursing Scholarship 31(3):215–220

Haig T H, Scott D A, Wickett L I 1986 The traditional zero point for an illness index with ratio properties. Medical Care 24(2):113–124

Haig T H, Scott D A, Stevens G B 1989 Measurement of the discomfort component of illness. Medical Care 27(3):280–287

Hajiro T, Nishimura K 2002 Minimal clinically significant difference in health status: the thorny path of health status measures? European Respiratory Journal 19:390–391

Haladyna T M, Downing S M 1988a A taxonomy of multiple-choice item – writing rules. Applied Measurement in Education 1:37–50

Haladyna T M, Downing S M 1988b The validity of a taxonomy of multiple-choice item – writing rules. Applied Measurement in Education 1:51–78

Hall J A, Epstein A M, McNeil B J 1989 Multidimensionality of health status in an elderly population. Medical Care 27:S168–S177

Hanita M 2000 Self-report measures of patient utility: should we trust them? Journal of Clinical Epidemiology 53:469–476

Harrison D A, McLaughlin M E 1993 Cognitive processes in self-report responses: test of item context effects in work attitude measures. Journal of Applied Psychology 78:129–140

Hawthorne G, Richardson J, Day N 2001 A comparison of the Assessment of Quality of Life (AQoL) with four other generic utility instruments. Annals of Medicine 33(5):358–370

Haynes R B, Devereaux P J, Guyatt G H 2002 Physicians' and patients' choices in evidence based practice. British Medical Journal 324:1350

Hays R D, Morales L S 2001 The RAND-36 measure of health-related quality of life. Annals of Medicine 33(5):350–357

Hays R D, Prince-Embury S, Chen H 1998 RAND-36 Health Status Inventory. Psychological Corp, San Antonio, TX

Hays W L 1973 Statistics for the social sciences, 2nd edn. Holt, Rinehart & Winston, New York

Hays W L 1981 Statistics for psychologists. Holt, Rinehart and Wilson, New York

Hays R D, Morales L S, Reise S P 2000 Item response theory and health outcomes measurements in the 21st century. Medical Care 38(9, suppl):II 28–42

Heady B, Wearing A W 1989 Personality, life events, and subjective well-being: towards a dynamic equilibrium model. Journal of Personality and Social Psychology 57:731–739

Heady B, Glowacki T, Holmstrom E et al 1985 Modelling change in PQoL. Social Indicators Research 17:267–298

Henson Robin K 2001 Understanding internal consistency reliability estimates: a conceptual primer on coefficient alpha. Measurement and Evaluation in Counseling and Development 34(3):177–189

Heyland K K, Guyyatt G, Cook D J et al 1998 Frequency and methodological rigor of quality of life assessments in the critical care literature. Critical Care Medicine 26(3):591–598

Higginson I J, Carr A J 2001 Measuring quality of life: using quality of life measures in the clinical setting. British Medical Journal 322:1297–1300

Hinkle D E, Oliver J D, Hinkle C A 1985 How large should the sample be? Part II – the one-sample case. Educational and Psychological Measurement 45:271–280

Hughes J E 1985 Depressive illness and lung cancer: depression before diagnosis. European Journal of Surgical Oncology 11:15–20

Hurny C, Bernhard J, Coates A et al 1996 Responsiveness of a single-item indicator versus a multi-item scale: assessment of emotional well-being in an international adjuvant breast cancer trial. Medical Care 34(3):234–248

Husted J A, Cook R J, Farewell V T et al 2000 Methods for assessing responsiveness: a critical review and recommendations. Journal of Clinical Epidemiology 53:459–468

Hyland M E 2002 Recommendations from quality of life scales are not simple. British Medical Journal 325:599

Jachuck S J, Brierley H, Jachuck S, Willcox P M 1982 The effect of hypotensive drugs on the quality of life. The Journal of the Royal College of General Practitioners 32(235):103–105

Jaeschke R, Singer J, Guyatt G H 1989 Measurement of health status: ascertaining the minimal clinically important difference. Controlled Clinical Trials 10:407–415

Jayasuriya R, Ruta D, Maitland H et al 1997 Patient perspectives of well-being: results of a study of outcome measurement in community nursing. Paper presented to 'Managing & Measuring Health Outcomes: from Policy to Practice', The Australian Health Outcomes Collaboration, Canberra, 31 October–1 November 1997

Jones P W 2002 Interpreting thresholds for a clinically significant change in health status in asthma and COPD. European Respiratory Journal 19(3):398–404

Juniper E F, Guyatt G H, Epstein R S et al 1992 Evaluation of impairment of health-related quality of life in asthma: development of a questionnaire for use in clinical trials. Thorax 47:76–83

Kahneman D 2000 Experienced utility and objective happiness: a moment-based approach. In: Kahneman D, Tversky A (eds) Choices, values and frames.

Cambridge University Press and the Russell Sage Foundation, New York, pp. 673–692

Kane R L 1997 Understanding health care outcomes research. Aspen, Gaithersburg, MD

Kaplan R M, Anderson J P 1988 A general health policy model: update and applications. Health Services Research 23(2):203–235

Kaplan R M, Ernst J A 1983 Do category rating scales produce biased preference weights for a health index? Medical Care XXI(2):193–207

Kaplan R M, Bush J W, Berry C C 1976 Health status: types of validity and the index of well being. Health Services Research 11(4):487–507

Kaplan R M, Bush J W, Berry C C 1979 Health status index: category rating versus magnitude estimation for measuring levels of well-being. Medical Care XVII(5):501–521

Kaplan R M, Anderson J P 1996 The general health policy model: an integrated approach. In: Spilker B (ed) Quality of life and pharmaeconomics in clinical trials, 2nd edn. Lippincott-Raven Publishers, Philadelphia, pp. 306–322

Kaplan R M, Anderson J P, Wu A W et al 1989 The quality of well-being scale. Medical Care 27(3):S27–S43

Kaplan R M, Feeny D, Revicki D A 1993 Methods for assessing relative importance in preference based outcome measures. Quality of Life Research 2(6):467–475

Kaplan S H, Kravitz R L, Greenfield S 2000 A critique of current uses of health status for the assessment of treatment effectiveness and quality of care. Medical Care 38(9, suppl):II 184–193

Kastrup M, Mezzich J E 2001 Quality of life: a dimension in multiaxial classification. European Archives of Psychiatry and Clinical Neuroscience 251 (suppl 2):II/32–II/37

Kazis L E, Anderson J J, Meena R F 1989 Effect sizes for interpreting changes in health status. Medical Care 27(3):S178–S189

Keller S D, Ware J E, Bentler P M et al 1998a Use of structural equation modeling to test the construct validity of the SF-36 health survey in ten countries: results from the IQoLA Project. Journal of Clinical Epidemiology 51(11):1179–1188

Keller S D, Ware J E, Gandek B et al 1998b Testing the equivalence of translations of widely used response choice labels: results from the IQOLA Project. Journal of Clinical Epidemiology 51(11):933–944

Kelley T L 1927 Interpretation of educational measurements. World Books, New York

Kennedy I 2003 Patients are experts in their own field: the interests of patients and healthcare professionals are intertwined. British Medical Journal 326:1276–1277

Kind D L, Rosser R 1988 The quantification of health. European Journal of Social Psychology 18:63–77

Kirshner B, Guyatt G 1985 A methodological framework for assessing health indices. Journal of Chronic Diseases 38:27–36

Kliempt P, Ruta D, McMurdo M 2000 Measuring the outcomes of care in older people: a non-critical review of patient-based measures. I. General health status and quality of life instruments. Reviews in Clinical Gerontology 10(1):33–42

Krabbe P F, Stouthard M, Essink-Bot M L et al 1999 The effect of adding a cognitive dimension to the EuroQol multiattribute health-status classification system. Journal of Clinical Epidemiology 52(4):293–301

Kurtin P S, Davies A R, Meyer K B et al 1992 Patient-based health status measures in outpatient dialysis. Medical Care 30(suppl):MS136–149

Lee C W, Chi K N 2000 The standard of reporting of health-related quality of life in clinical cancer trials. Journal of Clinical Epidemiology 53:451–458

Lenert L, Kaplan R M 2000 Validity and interpretation of preference-based measures of health-related quality of life. Medical Care 38(9, suppl):II 138–150

Leplège A, Rude N, Ecosse E et al 1997 Measuring quality of life from the point of view of HIV-positive subjects: the HIV-QL31. Quality of Life Research 6:585–594

Levi P 1987 If this is a man. Abacus, London

Liang M H 2000 Longitudinal construct validity: establishment of clinical meaning in patient evaluative instruments. Medical Care 38(9, suppl):II 84–90

Linacre J M 1995 KeyFIM – self-measuring score form. Rasch Measurement Transactions 9:453–454

Linacre J M 1996a True-score reliability or Rasch statistical validity? Rasch Measurement Transaction 9(4):455–456

Linacre J M 1996b The Rasch model cannot be 'disproved'! Rasch Measurement Transactions 10(3):512–514

Linacre J M 1997 KR-20 or Rasch reliability: which tells the 'truth'? Rasch Measurement Transactions 11(3):580–581

Linacre J M 1998 Rasch first or factor first? Rasch Measurement Transactions 11(4):603

Linacre J M 1999 Understanding (or misunderstanding?) the Rasch model. Rasch Measurement Transactions 13(3):706

Linacre J M 2002 What do infit and outfit, mean-square and standardized mean? Rasch Measurement Transactions 16(2):878

Linacre J M 2003a WINSTEPS Rasch measurement computer program. Chicago: Winsteps.com Downloaded from www.winsteps.com 11 June 2003

Linacre J M 2003b A user's guide to W I N S T E P S M I N I S T E P. Rasch-Model Computer Programs. Online. Available: www.winsteps.com 11 June 2003

Lipscomb J 1989 Time preference for health in cost-effectiveness analysis. Medical Care 27(3):S233–S253

Little P S, Williamson I, Warner G et al 1997 An open randomised trial of prescribing strategies for sore throat. British Medical Journal 314:722–727

Little P, Everitt H, Williamson I et al 2001 Observational study of effect of patient centredness and positive approach on outcomes of general practice consultations. British Medical Journal 323:20

Littlewood T J, Bajetta E, Nortier J W et al 2001 Effects of epoetin alfa on hematologic parameters and quality of life in cancer patients receiving nonplatinum chemotherapy: results of a randomized, double-blind, placebo-controlled trial. Journal of Clinical Oncology 19:2865–2874

Llewellyn-Thomas H, Sutherland H J, Tibshirani R et al 1984 Describing health states. Medical Care 22(6):543–552

Llewellyn-Thomas H A, Thiel E C, McGreal M J 1992 Cancer patients; evaluations of their current health states. Medical Decision Making 12:115–122

Loewenstein G F, Schkade D 1997 'Wouldn't it be nice? predicting future feelings'. Paper presented at the 1997 National Science Foundation Symposium on Eliciting Preferences. Online. Available: http://emlab.berkeley.edu/eml/nsf97/nsf97.html 16 July 2003

Lucas R E, Clark A E, Georgellis Y et al 2003 Reexamining adaptation and the set point model of happiness: reactions to changes in marital status. Journal of Personality and Social Psychology 84(3):527–539

Luce R D, Tukey J W 1964 Simultaneous conjoint measurement. Journal of Mathematical Psychology 1:1–27

Lumley T, McNamara T F 1995 Rater characteristics and rater bias: implications for training. Language-Testing 12(1):54–71

Lusardi M M, Smith E V 1997 Development of a scale to assess concern about falling and applications to treatment programs. Journal of Outcome Measurement 7(1):34–55

Lydick E, Epstein R 1996 Clinical significance of quality of life data. In: Spiker B (ed) Quality of life and pharmacoeconomics in clinical trials, 2nd edn. Lippincott-Raven Publishers, Philadelphia, New York, pp. 461–465

MacCallum R C, Austin J T 2000 Applications of structural equation modelling in psychological research. Annual Review of Psychology 51:201–226

McDowell I, Newell C 1996 Measuring health: a guide to rating scales and questionnaires, 2nd edn. Oxford University Press, New York

McHorney C A, Cohen A S 2000 Equating health status measures with item response theory: illustrations with functional status items. Medical Care 38(9, suppl):II 43–59

McHorney C A, Ware J J, Raczek A E 1993 The MOS 36-item short-form health survey (SF-36): II. Psychometric and clinical tests of validity in measuring physical and mental health constructs. Medical Care 31(3):247–263

McKinley R K, Manku-Scott T, Hastings A M et al 1997 Reliability and validity of a new measure of patient satisfaction with out of hours primary medical care in the united kingdom: development of a patient questionnaire. British Medical Journal 314:193

McNeil B J, Pauker S G, Sox H C et al 1982 On the elicitation of preferences for alternative therapies. New England Journal of Medicine 306:1259–1262

Machin D, Weeden S 1998 Suggestions for the presentation of quality of life data from clinical trials. Statistics in Medicine 17:711–724

Martin D P, Gilson B S, Bergner M et al 1976 The sickness impact profile: potential use of a health status instrument for physician training. Journal of Medical Education 51(11):942–944

Mason S, Hussain-Gambles M, Leese B et al 2003 Representation of South Asian people in randomised clinical trials: analysis of trials' data. British Medical Journal 326:1244–1245

Masters G N 1993 Undesirable item discrimination. Rasch Measurement Transactions 7(2):289

Mellers B A, Schwartz A, Cooke A D J 1998 Judgment and decison making. Annual Review of Psychology 49:447–477

Michell J 1997 Quantitative science and the definition of measurement in psychology. British Journal of Psychology 88(3):355–383

Min S K, Kim K I, Lee C I et al 2002 Development of the Korean versions of WHO quality of life scale and WHOQoL-BREF. Quality of Life Research 11(6):593–600

Moinpour C M, Sawyers T J, McKnight B et al 2000 Challenges posed by non-random missing quality of life data in an advanced-stage colorectal cancer clinical trial. Psycho-Oncology 9(4):340–354

Möller H J 2001 Methodological aspects in the assessment of severity of depression by the Hamilton Depression Scale. European Archives of Psychiatry and Clinical Neuroscience 251(suppl 2):II/13–II/20

Moser C, Kalton G 1979 Survey methods in social investigation, 2nd edn. Heinemann Educational Books, London

Muldoon M F, Barger S D, Flory J D et al 1998 What are quality of life measurements measuring? British Medical Journal 316(7130):542–545

Mulley A G 1989 Assessing patients; utilities. Medical Care 27:S269–S281

Mullin P A, Lohr K N, Bresnahan B W et al 2000 Applying cognitive design principles to formatting HRQOL instruments. Quality of Life Research 9(1):13–27

Nease R F 2000 Challenges in the validation of preference-based measures of health-related quality of life. Medical Care 38(9, suppl):II 155–159

Norman G 2003 Hi! How are you? Response shift, implicit theories and differing epistemologies. Quality of Life Research 12:239–249

Norman G R, Stratford P W, Regehr G 1997 Methodological problems in the retrospective computation of responsiveness to change: the lesson of Cronbach. Journal of Clinical Epidemiology 50(8):869–879

Norman G R, Sridhar F G, Guyatt G H et al 2001 Relation of distribution- and anchor-based approaches in interpretation of changes in health-related quality of life. Medical Care 39(10):1039–1047

Nortvedt M W, Riise T, Myhr K M, Nyland H I 2000 Performance of the SF-36, SF-12, and RAND-36 summary scales in a multiple sclerosis population. Medical Care 38(10):1022–1028

Nunnally J C 1978 Psychometric theory. McGraw-Hill, New York

Nunnally J C, Bernstein I H 1994 Psychometric Theory, 3rd edn. McGraw-Hill Series in Psychology, New York

O'Connor A M, Rostom A, Fiset V et al 1999a Decision aids for patients facing health treatment or screening decisions: systematic review. British Medical Journal 319:731–734

O'Connor R 1993 Issues in the measurement of health-related quality of life, Working Paper 30. NHMRC National Centre for Health Program Evaluation, Melbourne

O'Connor R 1995 Development of the health effects scale, Working Paper 43. NHMRC National Centre for Health Program Evaluation, Melbourne

O'Connor R 1996 Multi-centre clinical trial of instruments for assessing the disability support pension. For the Australian Government Health Service. Rod O'Connor & Associates P/L, Sydney

O'Connor R, Gibson C, Jenkins C, Mitchell C, Peters M 2000 Development of a new instrument for predicting adherence to asthma medication. World Congress on Lung Health, Florence, Italy

Osoba D 1994 Lessons learned from measuring health-related quality of life in oncology. Journal of Clinical Oncology 12:608–616

Osman L M, Godden D J, Friend J A R et al 1997 Quality of life and hospital re-admission in patients with chronic obstructive pulmonary disease. Thorax 52:67–71

Parducci A 1968 The relativism of absolute judgements. Scientific American 219:85–90

Patrick D L, Deyo R A 1989 Generic and disease-specific measures in assessing health status and quality of life. Medical Care 27(3):S217–S232

Patrick D L, Chiang Y-P 2000a Measurement of health outcomes in treatment effectiveness evaluations: conceptual and methodological challenges. Medical Care 38(9, suppl):II 14–27

Patrick D L, Chiang Y-P 2000b Postscript: the remaining questions. Medical Care 38(9, suppl):II 209–210

Patrick D L, Bush J W, Chen M M 1973 Methods for measuring levels of well-being for a health status index. Health Services Research 8(3):228–245

Perline R, Wright B D, Wainer H 1979 The Rasch model as additive conjoint measurement. Applied Psychological Measurement 3(2):237–255

Phillips R C, Lansky D J 1992 Outcomes management in heart valve replacement surgery: early experiences. Journal of Heart Valve Disease 1:42–50

Power M, Bullinger M, Harper A 1999 The World Health Organization WHOQoL-100: tests of the universality of quality of life in 15 different cultural groups worldwide. Health Psychology 18(5):495–505

Pugh-Clarke K, Koufaki P, Rowley V et al 2002 Improvement in quality of life of dialysis patients during six months of exercise. Edtna-Erca Journal 28(1):11–12

Raczek A E, Ware J E, Bjorner J B et al 1998 Comparison of Rasch and summated rating scales constructed from SF-36 physical functioning items in seven countries: results from the IQoLA Project. Journal of Clinical Epidemiology 51(11):1203–1214

Rasch G 1960 Probabilistic models for some intelligence and attainment tests. Danmarks Paedagogiske Institut, Copenhagen

Rasch G 1966 An item analysis which takes individual differences into account. British Journal of Mathematical and Statistical Psychology 19:49–57

Rasch G 1980 Probabilistic models for some intelligence and attainment tests, expanded edn. University of Chicago Press, Chicago

Read J L, Quinn R J, Berwick D M et al 1984 Preferences for health outcomes: comparison of assessment methods. Medical Decision Making 4(3):315–329

Redelmeier D A, Kahneman D 1996 Patients' memories of painful medical treatments: real-time and retrospective evaluations of two minimally invasive procedures. Pain 66:3–8

Redelmeier D A, Rozin P, Kahneman D 1993 Understanding patients' decisions: cognitive and emotional perspectives. JAMA 270(1):72–76

Ren X S, Kazis L 1998 Are patients capable of attributing functional impairments to specific diseases? American Journal of Public Health 88(5):837–838

Revicki D A 1989 Health related quality of life in the evaluation of medical therapy for chronic illness. Journal of Family Practice 29(4):377–380

Revicki D A, Cella D F 1997 Health status assessment for the twenty-first century: item response theory, item banking and computer adaptive testing. Quality of Life Research 6:595–600

Revicki D A, Osoba D, Fairclough D et al 2000 Recommendations on health-related quality of life research to support labeling and promotional claims in the United States. Quality of Life Research 9:887–900

Richardson J 1994 Cost utility analysis: what should be measured? Social Science & Medicine 39(1):7–21

Richardson J 1997 Critique and some recent contributions to the theory of cost utility analysis. Paper presented to 'Managing and Measuring Health Outcomes: from Policy to Practice'. Canberra, 31 October–1 November 1997

Ringdal G I, Jordhøy M S, Kaasa S 2003 Measuring quality of palliative care: Psychometric properties of the FAMCARE Scale. Quality of Life Research 12:167–176

Rosenkranz M A, Jackson D C, Dalton K M et al 2003 Affective style and in vivo immune response: neurobehavioral mechanisms. Proceedings of the National Academy of Sciences of the United States of America 100(19):11148–11152

Rothwell P M, McDowell Z, Wong C K et al 1997 Doctors and patients don't agree: cross sectional study of patients' and doctors' perceptions and assessments of disability in multiple sclerosis. British Medical Journal 314(7094):1580–1583

Rozin P, Nemeroff C 1990 The laws of sympathetic magic: a psychological analysis of similarity and contagion. In: Stigler J, Herdt G, Shweder RA (eds) Cultural psychology: essays of comparative human development. Cambridge University Press, New York, NY

Rudner L 1998 Item banking. Practical assessment, research & evaluation 6(4). ERIC Clearinghouse on Assessment and Evaluation. Online. Available: http://ericae.net

Ruta D A, Garratt A M, Russell I T 1999 Patient centered assessment of quality of life for patients with four common conditions. Quality in Health Care 8(1):22–29

Ryan M, Farrar S 2000 Using conjoint analysis to elicit preferences for health care. British Medical Journal 320:1530–1533

Ryan R M, Deci E L 2001 On happiness and human potentials: a review of research on hedonic and eudaimonic well-being. Annual Review of Psychology 52:141–166

Sackett D L, Torrance G W 1978 The utility of different health states as perceived by the general public. Journal of Chronic Diseases 31:697–704

Sade R M 2001 Deceiving insurance companies: new expression of an ancient tradition. Annals of Thoracic Surgery 72:1449–1453

Saigal C, Gornbein J, Litwin M S 2001 Patient utilities for complications do not predict treatment choice in men with clinically localized prostate cancer. Journal of Clinical Outcomes Management 8(8)

Sales E 2003 Family burden and quality of life. Quality of Life Research 12(suppl 1):33–41

Salzberger T 2000 Intercultural construct validity in emic and etic research. Proceedings of the 2000 Multicultural Marketing Conference (AMS), 2000 September 17–20, Grand Stanford Harbor View Hotel, Kowloon, Hong Kong, PRC

Salzberger T 2002 The illusion of measurement: Rasch versus 2-PL. Rasch Measurement Transactions 16(2):882

Samsa G 2001 How should the minimum important difference for a health-related quality-of-life instrument be estimated? Medical Care 39(10):1037–1038

Sanders C, Egger M, Donovan J et al 1998 Reporting on quality of life in randomised controlled trials: bibliographic study. British Medical Journal 317:1191–1194

Saxena S, Carlson D, Billington R et al 2001 The WHO quality of life assessment instrument (WHOQoL-Bref): the importance of its items for cross-cultural research. Quality of Life Research 10:711–721

Schmitt N, Chan D, Sacco J M et al 1999 Correlates of person fit and effect of person fit on test validity. Applied Psychological Measurement 23(1):41–53

Schneiderman N, Antoni M H, Saab P G et al 2001 Health psychology: psychosocial and biobehavioral aspects of chronic disease management. Annual Review of Psychology 52:555–580

Schumacker R E, Linacre J M 1996 Factor analysis and Rasch analysis. Rasch Measurement Transactions 9(4):470

Schwarz N, Strack F 1991 Evaluating one's life: a judgement model of subjective well-being. In: Strack F, Argyle M, Schwarz N (eds) Subjective well-being: an interdisciplinary perspective. Pergamon Press, Oxford, pp. 27–48

Sen S S, Gupchup G V, Thomas J 1999 Selecting among health-related quality-of-life instruments. American Journal of Health-System Pharmacy 56:Oct 1

Shavelson R J 1988 Statistical Reasoning for the behavioural sciences, 2nd edn. Allyn and Bacon, Inc., Boston

Shumaker S A, Ellis S, Naughton M 1997 Assessing health-related quality of life in HIV disease: key measurement issues. Quality of Life Research 6:475–480

Silberfeld M, Rueda S, Krahn M et al 2002 Content validity for dementia of three generic preference based health related quality of life instruments. Quality of Life Research: an International Journal of Quality of Life Aspects of Treatment, Care and Rehabilitation 11(1):71–79

Simes R J, Greatorex V, Gebski V J 1998 Practical approaches to minimize problems with missing quality of life data. Statistics in Medicine (5–7):725–737

Skeel R T 1989 Quality of life assessment in cancer and clinical trials: it's time to check up. Journal of the National Cancer Institute 81:72–73

Sloan J A, Loprinzi C L, Kuross S A et al 1998 Randomized comparison of four tools measuring overall quality of life in patients with advanced cancer. Journal of Clinical Oncology 16:3662–3673

Sloan J A, Aaronson N, Cappelleri J C et al 2002a Assessing the clinical significance of single items relative to summated scores. Mayo Clinic Proceedings 77(5):479–487

Sloan J A, Cella D, Frost M et al 2002b Assessing clinical significance in measuring oncology patient quality of life: introduction to the symposium, content overview, and definition of terms. Mayo Clinic Proceedings 77(4):367–370

Smith E V 2002 Detecting and evaluating the impact of multidimensionality using item fit statistics and principal component analysis of residuals. Journal of Applied Measurement 3(2):205–231

Smith R M 1992 Applications of Rasch measurement. JAM Press, Maple Grove, MN

Smith R M 1996 A comparison of methods for determining dimensionality in Rasch measurement. Structural Equation Modelling 3(1):25–40

Smith R M 2000 Fit analysis in latent trait measurement models. Journal of Applied Measurement 1(2):199–218

Smith R M, Miao C Y 1994 Assessing unidimensionality for Rasch measurement. In: Wilson M (ed) Objective measurement: theory into practice, vol 2. Ablex, Norwood, NJ

Spector P F 1976 Choosing response categories for summated rating scales. Journal of Applied Psychology 61(3):374–375

Stahl J 1990 Lost in the dimensions. Rasch Measurement Transactions 4:4

StatSoft Inc 1999 Electronic Statistics Textbook. OK: StatSoft, Tulsa. Online. Available: http://www.statsoft.com/textbook/stathome.html

Steinhauser K E, Clipp E C, Tulsky J A 2002 Evolution in measuring the quality of dying. Journal of Palliative Medicine 5(3):407–414

Stenner J 2001 The necessity of construct theory. Rasch Measurement Transactions 15(1):804–805

Stevens S S 1946 On the theory of measurement. Science 103:667–680

Stevens S S 1972 Psychophysics. In: Eysenck H J, Arnold W J, Meih R (eds) Encyclopaedia of psychology. Fontana/Collins.

Stevens S S, Galanter E H 1957 Ratio scales and category scales for a dozen perceptual continua. Journal of Experimental psychology 54(6):377–411

Stewart A L, Napoles-Springer A 2000 Health-related quality-of-life assessments in diverse population groups in the United States. Medical Care 38(9, suppl):II 102–124

Stiggelbout A M, de Haes J C 2001 Patient preference for cancer therapy: an overview of measurement approaches. Journal of Clinical Oncology 19(1):220–230

Streiner D L, Norman G R 1996 Health measurement scales, a practical guide to their development and use, 2nd edn. Oxford Medical Publications, Oxford

Sutherland H J, Dunn V, Boyd N F 1983 Measurement of values for states of health with linear analog scales. Medical Decision Making 3:479–487

Switzer G E, Wisniewski S R, Belle S H et al 1999 Selecting, developing, and evaluating research instruments. Social Psychiatry and Psychiatric Epidemiology 34(8):399–409

Taft C, Karlsson J, Sullivan M 2001a Do SF-36 summary component scores accurately summarize subscale scores? Quality of Life Research 10(5):395–404

Taft C, Karlsson J, Sullivan M 2001b Do SF-36 summary component scores accurately summarize subscale scores? Reply. Quality of Life Research 10(5):415–420

Tanaka T, Gotay C C 1998 Physicians' and medical students' perspectives on patients' quality of life. Academic Medicine 73:1003–1005

Temkin N R, Dikmen S, Machamer J et al 1989 General versus disease-specific measures. Medical Care 27(3):S44–S53

Testa M A 2000 Interpretation of quality-of-life outcomes: issues that affect magnitude-and meaning. Medical Care 38(9, suppl):II 166–174

Terwee C B, Dekker F W, Wiersinga W M et al 2003 On assessing responsiveness of health-related quality of life instruments: guidelines for instrument evaluation. Quality of Life Research 12:349–362

Thomee R, Grimby G, Wright B D et al 1995 Rasch analysis of visual analog scale measurements before and after treatment of patellofemoral pain syndrome in women. Scandinavian Journal of Rehabilitation Medicine 27(3):145–151

Thompson B 1995 Stepwise regression and stepwise discriminant analysis need not apply here: a guidelines editorial. Educational and Psychological Measurement 55(4):525–534

Thumboo J, Fong K Y, Chan S P et al 2002 The equivalence of English and Chinese SF-36 versions in bilingual Singapore Chinese. Quality of Life Research 11(5):495–503

Till J E 1994 Measuring quality of life: apparent benefits, potential concerns. Canadian Journal of Oncology 4(1):243–248

Toops H A 1944 The criterion. Educational and Psychological Measurement 4:271–297

Torrance G W 1976 Social preference for health status. Socio-economic Planning Sciences 10:129–136

Torrance G W 1986 Measurement of health state utilities for economic appraisal. Journal of Health Economics 5:1–30

Torrance G W 1987 Utility approach to measuring health-related quality of life. Journal of Chronic Diseases 40:593–600

Torrance G W, Feeny D 1989 Utilities and quality-adjusted life years. International Journal of Technology Assessment in Health Care 5:559–575

Torrance G W, Thomas W H, Sackett D L 1972 A utility maximisation model for evaluation of health care programs. Health Services Research 7:118–133

Torrance G W, Boyle M H, Horwood S P 1982 Application of multi attribute utility theory to measure social preference for health states. Operations Research 30:1043–1069

Troxel A B, Fairclough D L, Curran D et al 1998 Statistical analysis of quality of life with missing data in cancer clinical trials. Statistics in Medicine 17:653–666

Tsevat J 2000 What do utilities measure? Medical Care 38(9, suppl):II 160–165

Tsevat J, Dawson N V, Matchar D B 1990 Assessing quality of life and preference in the seriously ill using utility theory. Journal of Clinical Epidemiology 43:735–775

Tsuji T, Liu M, Sonoda S et al 2000 The stroke impairment assessment set: its internal consistency and predictive validity. Archives of Physical Medicine and Rehabilitation 81:863–868

Tversky A, Kahneman D 1981 The framing of decisions and the psychology of choice. Science 211:453–458

Uttaro T, Lehman A 1999 Graded response modeling of the quality of life interview. Evaluation and Program Planning 22:41–52

VanderZee K, Buunk B, DeRuiter J et al 1996 Social comparison and the subjective well-being of cancer patients. Basic and Applied Social Psychology 18(4):453–468

Velikova G, Brown J M, Smith A B et al 2002 Computer-based quality of life questionnaires may contribute to doctor-patient interactions in oncology. British Journal of Cancer 86(1):51–59

Verkerk M A, Busschbach J J V, Karssing E D 2001 Health-related quality of life research and the capability approach of Amartya Sen. Quality of Life Research: an International Journal of Quality of Life Aspects of Treatment, Care and Rehabilitation 10(1):49–55

Von Neumann J, Morgenstern O 1953 The theory of games and economic behaviour. Wiley, New York

Waldron D, O'Boyle C A, Kearney M et al 1999 Quality-of-life measurement in advanced cancer: assessing the individual. Journal of Clinical Oncology 17(11):3603–3611

Walker W R, Skowronski J J, Thompson C P 2003 Life is pleasant – and memory helps to keep it that way! Review of General Psychology (2):203–210

Ware J E 1993 SF-36 Health survey manual and interpretation guide. The Health Institute, New England Medical Centre, Boston

Ware J E, Sherbourne C D 1992 The MOS 36-item short-form health survey (SF-36) I. Conceptual framework and item selection. Medical Care 30(6):473–481

Ware J E, Keller S D 1996 Interpreting general health measures. In: Spilker B (ed) Quality of life and pharmacoeconomics in clinical trials, 2nd edn. Lippincott-Raven Publishers, Philadelphia, pp. 445–460

Ware J E, Kosinski M 2001 Interpreting SF-36 summary health measures: a response. Quality of Life Research 10(5):405–413

Ware J E, Davies-Avery A, Stewart A L 1978 The measurement and meaning of patient satisfaction. Health and Medical Care Services Review 1:2–15

Ware J E, Kosinski M, Keller S D 1996 A 12-item short form health survey: construction of scales and preliminary tests of reliability and validity. Medical Care 34(3):220–233

Ware J E, Bjomer J B, Kosinski M 2000 Practical implications of item response theory and computerized adaptive testing: a brief summary of ongoing studies of widely used headache impact scales. Medical Care 38(9, suppl):II 73–83

Watten R G, Vassend D, Myhrer T et al 1997 Personality factors and somatic symptoms. European Journal of Personality 11:57–68

Weinberger M, Samsa G P, Hanlon J T et al 1991 An evaluation of a brief health status measure in elderly veterans. Journal of the American Geriatrics Society 39(7):691–694

Weiner E A, Stewart B J 1984 Assessing individuals. Little Brown, Boston

Wilkin D, Hallam L, Doggett M 1993 Measures of need and outcome for primary health care. Oxford Medical Publications, Oxford

Wolfe F, Kong S X 1999 Rasch analysis of the Western Ontario MacMaster questionnaire (WOMAC) in 2205 patients with osteoarthritis, rheumatoid arthritis, and fibromyalgia. Annals of the Rheumatic Diseases 58(9):563–568

Wolinsky F D, Wyrwich K W, Nienaber N A et al 1998 Generic versus disease-specific health status measures. An example using coronary artery disease and congestive heart failure patients. Evaluation and the Health Professions 21(2):216–243

Wood-Dauphinee S 1999 Assessing quality of life in clinical research: from where have we come and where are we going? Journal of Clinical Epidemiology 52(4):355–363

World Health Organization 1947 Constitution of the World Health Organization. World Health Organization, New York

Wright B D 1988 Georg Rasch and measurement. Rasch Measurement Transactions 2(3):25–32

Wright B D 1992 What is the 'right' test length? Rasch Measurement Transactions 6(1):205

Wright B D 1994 Where do dimensions come from? Rasch Measurement Transactions 7(4):325

Wright B D 1996 Local dependency, correlations and principal components. Rasch Measurement Transactions 10(3):509–511

Wright B D 1997a Fundamental measurement for outcome evaluation. Physical medicine and rehabilitation. State of the Art Reviews 11(2):261–288

Wright B D 1997b Fundamental measurement. Rasch Measurement Transactions 11(2):558

Wright B D 1999 Fundamental measurement for psychology. In: Embretson S E, Hershberger S L (eds) The new rules of measurement: what every educator and psychologist should know. Lawrence Erlbaum Associates, Hillsdale, NJ

Wright B D, Tennant A 1996 Sample size again. Rasch Measurement Transactions 9(4):468

Wright J G 2000 Evaluating the outcome of treatment. Shouldn't we be asking patients if they are better? Journal of Clinical Epidemiology 53(6):549–553

Wrosch C, Scheier M F 2003 Personality and quality of life: the importance of optimism and goal adjustment. Quality of Life Research 12(suppl 1):59–72

Wu A W 2000 Quality-of-life assessment in clinical research: application in diverse populations. Medical Care 38(9, suppl):II 130–137

Wyrwich K W, Wolinsky F D 2000 Identifying meaningful intra-individual change standards for health-related quality of life measures. Journal of Evaluation in Clinical Practice 6(1):39–49

Wyrwich K W, Tierney W M, Wolinsky F D 2002 Using the standard error of measurement to identify important changes on the Asthma Quality of Life Questionnaire. Quality of Life Research 11:1–7

Yardley J K, Rice R W 1991 The relationship between mood and subjective well-being. Social Indicators Research 24:101–111

Yu C L M, Fielding R, Chan C L W 2003 The mediating role of optimism on post-radiation quality of life in nasopharyngeal carcinoma. Quality of Life Research 12:41–51

Zurawski R M 1998 Making the most of exams: procedures for item analysis. The National Teaching and Learning Forum. 7(6) Online. Available: http://www.ntlf.com/html/pi/9811/toc.htm 7 Nov 2003

Bibliography

Agresti A, Finlay B 1997 Statistical methods for the social sciences, 3rd edn. Prentice Hall, Upper Saddle River, NJ

Anastasi A, Urbina S 1996 Psychological testing, 7th edn. Prentice Hall, Upper Saddle River, NJ

Bowling A 1998 Measuring health: a review of quality of life measurement scales, 2nd edn. Open University Press, Buckingham

Cohen R J, Swerdlik M E 1999 Psychological testing and assessment. An introduction to tests and measurement, 4th edn. Mayfield Publishing Company, London

Dimsdale J, Baum A (eds) 1995 Quality of life in behavioural research. Lawrence Erlbaum Associates, New York, NY

Nunnally J C, Bernstein I H 1994 Psychometric theory, 3rd edn. McGraw-Hill Series in Psychology, New York, NY

Rust R, Golombok S 1999 Modern psychometrics. The science of psychological assessment, 2nd edn. Routledge, London

Spilker B (ed) 1996 Quality of life and pharmacoeconomics in clinical trials, 2nd edn. Lippincott-Raven, Philadelphia

Streiner D L, Norman G R 1996 Health measurement scales, a practical guide to their development and use, 2nd edn. Oxford Medical Publications, Oxford

Wilkin D, Hallam L, Doggett M A 1993 Measures of need and outcome for primary healthcare. Oxford University Press, Oxford

Index

Note: Page references in *italics* indicate figures and boxed material, abbreviations used in this index are the same as those listed on pages xv–xvi.

clinical validity, Sickness Impact
Profile, 174
clinician-based anchors, 207–208
'clinimetric global ratings', 78
coefficient alpha, 125–126
cognitive evaluation, 29–34
communication styles, 212
comparison studies, known-group, 58
computer adaptive testing (CAT),
153–155
computer-based tests, 44
conduct quantitative item analysis,
121–126, 130
confidence intervals, 101–102
confirmatory factor analysis (CFA),
63, 80
confusion scales, 71
conjoint measurement theory, 136–137
see also Rasch analysis
consistency, 200
internal, 95–97, 109
constructs, 11, 40–41, *41*, 157
cultural influences, 213
evaluation, 194–195, 196
interval properties, 134–138, 161
measurement, 46–47
validity, 53–54, 177–178
construct validity, 53–54, 177–178
consultations, GP, 8
content validity, 67
contraction bias, 72
convergent validity, 49, 58
Sickness Impact Profile, 173–174
coping mechanisms, 212
correlation, 63–66, 67–68
coefficients, 95
Pearson Product-Moment *see*
Pearson Product-Moment
Correlation
correlational studies, 58–59
correlation coefficient, 95
cost-utility analysis (CUA), 19
criteria identification, 42–48
practical needs, 42–45
computer-based, 44
interviewer *vs.* self-administered,
43–44
meaningfulness, 45
outputs, 44
size/time, 42–43
test development, 45–47, 48, 117
content, 45–46
forming/scaling, 46
psychometric properties, 46–47
validity, 46–47

criteria specification, *41*, 41–42
criterion measures
anchors, 208
benefits, 85–87
criteria specification, *41*, 41–42
global ratings, 84–87, 89
standard error of measurement
(SEM), 101–103
test evaluation, 197
validity, 59–61, 195, 200
visual analogue scales, *86*, 160
see also criteria identification
Cronbach's Alpha, 96–97, 102, 109
cross-cultural application of measures,
27, 202, 211–214, 220, 226
cultural issues
affect (mood) and health *vs.*, 27
cross-cultural application of
measures, 27, 202, 211–214,
220, 226
pan-cultural measures, 213
trans-cultural tests, 212–213

D

databases, 45
data, problems, 218–222, 227
'decision utility', 32
dementia, 56
descriptive validity, 57, 62, 174
descriptors, *87*
dichotomous model, 147, *147*, 232
differential group prediction, 58
differential item functioning (DIF),
155–156
dimension scores, 44
direct reporting, 78–79
disability, work-related *see* work-
related disability
discriminant capacity, 171
discriminant validity, 49, 58, 173–174
disease-specific measures, 16–18
distribution-based methods, 209–210
distribution, bivariate, 63
dynamic measures, 223–225, 227

E

elderly people, 10, 56–57
end-point definition, 74–75, 214
EORTC QLQ-C30, 7

W

'weighting systems', 85
'Well Life expectancy', 177
Weschler Adult Intelligence Scale
(WAIS), 97
Western Ontario MacMaster
Osteoarthritis Questionnaire
(WOMAC), 158
WHOQoL, 213
wording determination, 118–121,
122, 129

'Work Ability Tables', 41, 47–48, 122,
123, 126–127, 127
work-related disability, 41, 47–48,
122, 123
World Health Organization
definition of health, 2
Quality of Life (WHOQoL), 213

Z

zero point, 75